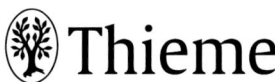

Direct Diagnosis in Radiology

Cardiac Imaging

Claus D. Claussen, MD
Professor of Radiology
Chairman
Department of Diagnostic and Interventional Radiology
Eberhard-Karls-University of Tübingen
Tübingen, Germany

Stephan Miller, MD
Professor of Radiology
Chief attending
Department of Diagnostic and Interventional Radiology
Eberhard-Karls-University of Tübingen
Tübingen, Germany

Reimer Riessen, MD
Professor of Internal Medicine
Director of the Medical Intensive Care Unit
Department of Medicine
Eberhard-Karls-University of Tübingen
Tübingen, Germany

Michael Fenchel, MD
Department of Diagnostic and Interventional Radiology
Eberhard-Karls-University of Tübingen
Tübingen, Germany

Ulrich Kramer, MD
Department of Diagnostic and Interventional Radiology
Eberhard-Karls-University of Tübingen
Tübingen, Germany

257 Illustrations

Thieme
Stuttgart · New York

Library of Congress
Cataloging-in-Publication

Herz. English.
    Cardiac imaging/Claus D. Claussen ... [et al.];
    translated by Terry Telger ; illustrated by
    Rose Baumann, Markus Voll, and Karl Wesker.
        p. ; cm.
    Includes bibliographical references and
    index.
    ISBN 978-3-13-145111-8 (TPS, rest of the
    world : alk. paper) –
    ISBN 978-1-60406-014-0 (TPN, the
    Americans : alk. paper) 1. Heart–Imaging–
    Handbooks, manuals, etc. 2. Heart–
    Diseases–Diagnosis–Handbooks, manuals,
    etc. I. Claussen, Claus, 1945- II. Title.
        [DNLM: 1. Diagnostic Techniques,
    Cardiovascular–Handbooks. 2. Diagnostic
    Imaging–Handbooks. 3. Heart Diseases–
    diagnosis–Handbooks. WG 39 H582 2007]
    RC683.5.I42H4713 2007
    616.1'207575–dc22   2007023540

This book is an authorized and revised transla-
tion of the German edition published and
copyrighted 2007 by Georg Thieme Verlag,
Stuttgart, Germany. Title of the German edition: Pareto-Reihe Radiologie: Herz.

Translated by Terry Telger, Fort Worth,
Texas, US

Illustrated by Rose Baumann, Schriesheim,
Germany; Markus Voll, Munich,
and Karl Wesker, Berlin (Prometheus).

© 2008 Georg Thieme Verlag KG
Rüdigerstrasse 14, 70469 Stuttgart, Germany
http://www.thieme.de
Thieme New York, 333 Seventh Avenue,
New York, NY 10001, USA
http://www.thieme.com

Cover design: Thieme Publishing Group
Typesetting by Ziegler + Müller,
Kirchentellinsfurt, Germany
Printed by APPL, aprinta Druck,
Wemding, Germany

ISBN 978-3-13-145111-8
(TPS, Rest of World)
ISBN 978-1-60406-014-0
(TPN, The Americas)   1 2 3 4 5 6

Important note: Medicine is an ever-chang-
ing science undergoing continual development. Research and clinical experience are
continually expanding our knowledge, in particular our knowledge of proper treatment
and drug therapy. Insofar as this book men-
tions any dosage or application, readers may
rest assured that the authors, editors, and
publishers have made every effort to ensure
that such references are in accordance with
**the state of knowledge at the time of pro-
duction of the book.**

Nevertheless, this does not involve, imply, or
express any guarantee or responsibility on
the part of the publishers in respect to any
dosage instructions and forms of applications
stated in the book. **Every user is requested to
examine carefully** the manufacturers' leaflets accompanying each drug and to check, if
necessary in consultation with a physician or
specialist, whether the dosage schedules
mentioned therein or the contraindications
stated by the manufacturers differ from the
statements made in the present book. Such
examination is particularly important with
drugs that are either rarely used or have been
newly released on the market. Every dosage
schedule or every form of application used is
entirely at the user's own risk and responsibility. The authors and publishers request every
user to report to the publishers any discrepan-
cies or inaccuracies noticed. If errors in this
work are found after publication, errata will
be posted at www.thieme.com on the product
description page.

Some of the product names, patents, and registered designs referred to in this book are in
fact registered trademarks or proprietary
names even though specific reference to this
fact is not always made in the text. Therefore,
the appearance of a name without designation
as proprietary is not to be construed as a rep-
resentation by the publisher that it is in the
public domain.

Contents

Contents

10 Diseases of the Great Vessels
U. Kramer

11 Standard Views of the Heart
S. Miller

12 Appendix
S. Miller

3D	Three-dimensional	**ESV**	End-systolic volume
AHA	American Heart Association	**FDG**	Fluoro-18-deoxyglucose
ALCA	Anomalous origin of left coronary artery	**FLAIR**	Fluid-attenuated inversion recovery
AMI	Acute myocardial infarction	**FSE**	Fast spin echo
A-P	Anterior-posterior	**GE**	Gradient echo
ARCA	Anomalous origin of right coronary artery	**HASTE**	Half-Fourier single-shot turbo spin echo
ARVC	Arrhythmogenic right ventricular cardiomyopathy	**HCM**	Hypertrophic cardio-myopathy
ARVD	Arrhythmogenic right ventricular dysplasia	**HLHS**	Hypoplastic left heart syndrome
ASD	Atrial septal defect	**HOCM**	Hypertrophic obstructive cardiomyopathy
AV	Atrioventricular	**HU**	Hounsfield unit
AVR	Aortic valve reconstruction	**ICD**	Implantable cardioverter-defibrillator
AVSD	Atrioventricular septal defect	**ILNC**	Isolated left ventricular noncompaction
CHD	Coronary heart disease	**IR**	Inversion recovery
CK	Creatine kinase	**IVUS**	Intravascular ultrasound
CMV	Cytomegalovirus	**LA**	Left atrium, left atrial
CNS	Central nervous system	**LAD**	Left anterior descending artery
COPD	Chronic obstructive pulmonary disease	**LBBB**	Left bundle branch block
CT	Computed tomography, computed tomogram	**LCA**	Left coronary artery
		LCX	Left circumflex artery
CTA	CT angiography	**LV**	Left ventricle, left ventricular
CTR	Cardiothoracic ratio		
CVC	Central venous catheter	**LVOT**	Left ventricular outflow tract
DAo	Double aortic arch		
DCM	Dilated cardiomyopathy	**MAPCA**	Major aortopulmonary collateral arteries
DD	Differential diagnosis		
DORV	Double-outlet right ventricle	**MIP**	Maximum intensity projection
DSA	Digital subtraction angiography	**MPR**	Multiplanar reconstruction
DTPA	Diethylenetriaminepenta-acetic acid	**MRA**	Magnetic resonance angiography
ECA	External carotid artery	**MRI**	Magnetic resonance imaging
ECG	Electrocardiography	**MVP**	Mitral valve prolapse
EDV	End-diastolic volume	**NYHA**	New York Heart Association
EF	Ejection fraction		
ESC	European Society of Cardiology	**P-A**	Posterior-anterior
		PA	Pulmonary artery

PC	Pulmonary capillary	**RVOT**	Right ventricular outflow tract
PDA	Patent ductus arteriosus		
PET	Positron emission tomography	**SPECT**	Single photon emission computed tomography
PFO	Patent foramen ovale	**SSD**	Shaded surface display
PI	Pulmonary insufficiency	**SSFP**	Steady-state free precession
PRIND	Prolonged reversible ischemic neurologic defect	**TAPVC**	Total anomalous pulmonary venous connection
PS	Pulmonary stenosis		
PT	Pulmonary trunk	**TEE**	Transesophageal echocardiography
PTCA	Percutaneous trans-coronary angioplasty	**TGA**	Transposition of the great arteries
PTFE	Polytetrafluoroethylene (Teflon)	**TI**	Tricuspid insufficiency
RAo	Retroesophageal right aortic arch	**TIA**	Transient ischemic attack
		TOF	Tetralogy of Fallot
RAO	Right anterior oblique (projection)	**TOS**	Thoracic outlet syndrome
		TS	Tricuspid stenosis
RBBB	Right bundle branch block	**TSE**	Turbo spin echo
RCM	Restrictive cardiomyopathy	**TTE**	Transthoracic echocardiography
RCA	Right coronary artery	**VOA**	Valve opening area
RCX	Circumflex branch of the left coronary artery	**VRT**	Volume rendering technique
RV	Right ventricle, right ventricular	**VSD**	Ventricular septal defect
		WPW	Wolff–Parkinson–White

Definition

▶ **Epidemiology**
Widespread in Western industrialized countries • Overall incidence increases with life expectancy • Prevalence approximately 4% • Present in approximately 5–10% of the male population • More common in males than in females (4:1).

▶ **Etiology, pathophysiology, pathogenesis**
Endothelial damage from "atherogenic risk factors" • Formation of atheromatous plaques • Reduction of luminal diameter (becomes critical at 70% narrowing) • Diminished coronary flow reserve.
Risk factors: Hyperlipoproteinemia, hypercholesterolemia, nicotine misuse, diabetes mellitus, arterial hypertension, obesity, familial disposition.

Imaging Signs

▶ **Modality of choice**
Invasive coronary angiography.

▶ **Chest radiograph findings**
Findings depend on the severity of the disease • Cardiopulmonary findings are initially normal • In severe cases LV enlargement, pulmonary venous congestion, and/or pleural effusion is seen.

▶ **Echocardiographic findings**
(Stress-induced) LV dysfunction (regional hypo- or akinesia) • LV dilatation may precede dilatation of the LA, depending on disease severity • Secondary mitral insufficiency • Chronic congestion leads to pulmonary vein dilatation.

▶ **Nuclear medicine and PET findings**
Detection and quantification of myocardial perfusion defects and dysfunction.

▶ **CT findings**
Calcified plaques (calcium scoring) and soft plaques on multidetector CT angiography • Coronary stenoses • Signs of left-sided heart failure.

▶ **MRI findings**
Same as echocardiography • MRA may show coronary stenoses • Decreased myocardial perfusion in response to pharmacologic stress (adenosine) • Myocardial infarction is detected by delayed contrast enhancement of the myocardial scar after gadolinium-DTPA administration (IR GE sequence).

▶ **Invasive diagnostic procedures**
Coronary angiography: One or more stenotic coronary arteries • *IVUS:* More accurately delineates plaques and stenoses.

Fig. 1.1 P-A chest radiograph in CHD. Marked enlargement of the LV due to heart failure, and increased pulmonary vascular markings due to chronic pulmonary venous congestion. A goiter with tracheal narrowing was noted as an incidental finding.

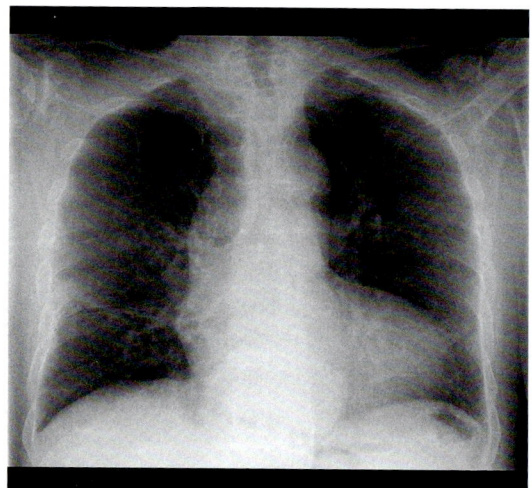

Fig. 1.2 High-grade stenosis of the LCX shown by coronary angiography.

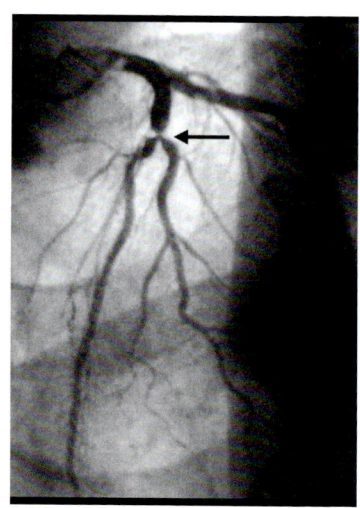

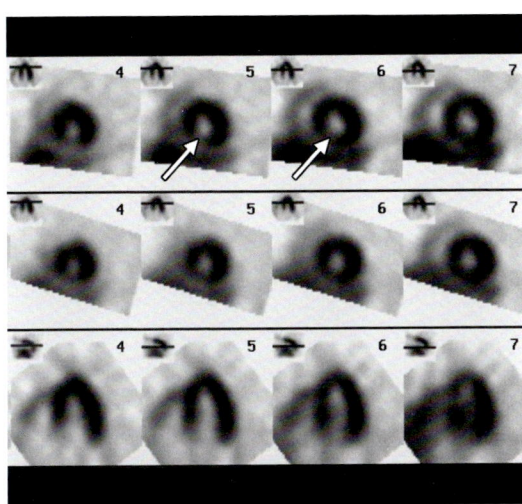

Fig. 1.3 Myocardial scintigraphy. An apical perfusion defect (arrow).

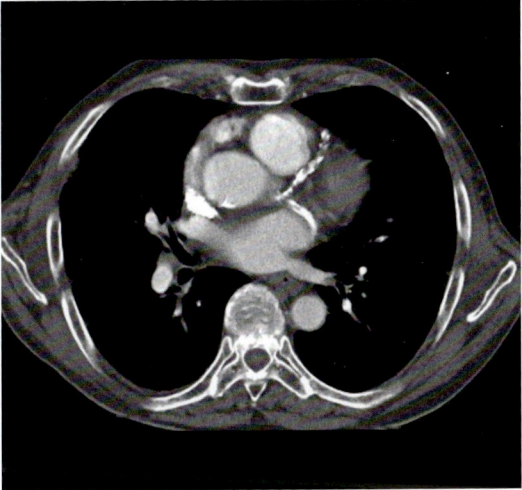

Fig. 1.4 Multi-detector CT. Diffuse sclerosis of the LCA.

Fig. 1.5 Coronary stent in a 65-year-old woman with known CHD. Curved MPR of a stent in segment 3 of the right coronary artery shows no morphologic evidence of in-stent restenosis.

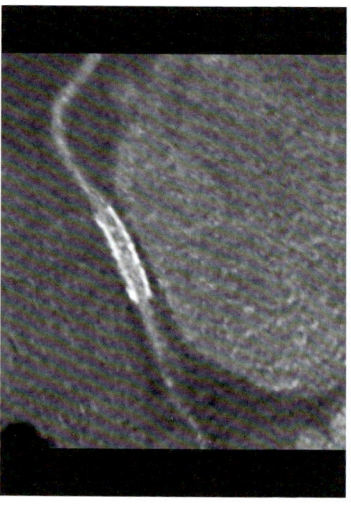

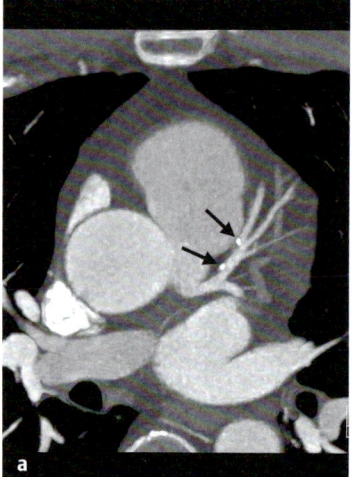

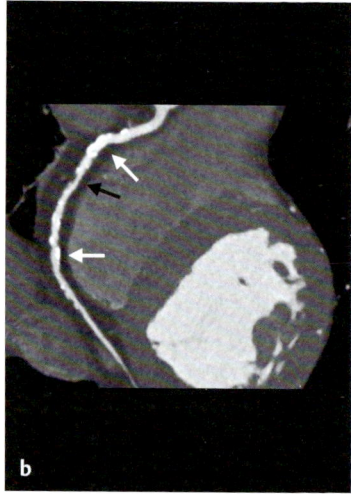

Fig. 1.6 a, b Coronary plaque in a 56-year-old man with nonspecific chest discomfort. The patient had no ECG abnormalities and an echocardiogram also showed normal findings. Coronary status was investigated by cardiac CT. Two mildly stenosing mixed plaques (arrows) are seen in segments 6 and 8 of the LAD artery (**a**). Curved MPR of the right coronary artery shows moderately stenosing calcified plaques (white arrows) in segments 2 and 3 and a moderately stenosing soft plaque (black arrow) in segment 2 (**b**).

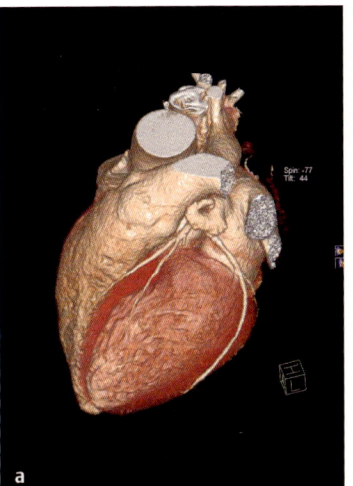

Fig. 1.7 a, b Coronary status in a 60-year-old woman with a familial disposition for CHD, current dyspnea, and nonspecific ECG changes. Cardiac CT was done to exclude CHD, and VRT was used for three-dimensional cardiac imaging. This technique is useful for demonstrating findings (**a**), but the actual diagnosis should always rely on thin reconstructed slices or MPRs (see below). Curved MPRs of normal coronary vessels (**b**). Left panel: RCA; center panel: LAD; right panel: LCX.

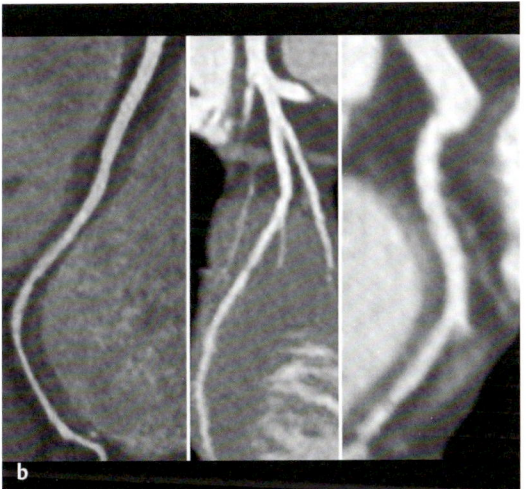

Clinical Aspects

▶ **Typical presentation**
Angina pectoris • Exertional dyspnea • Heart failure • Cardiac arrhythmias.

▶ **Treatment options**
Medical treatment for ischemic heart disease and cardiac insufficiency • Interventional (PTCA, stent implantation) or surgical (aortocoronary bypass) myocardial revascularization.

▶ **Course and prognosis**
Depend on the location and degree of coronary stenosis, myocardial ischemia, LV function (EF), and continued exposure to risk factors • *Complications:* Arrhythmias, myocardial infarction, left-sided heart failure, sudden cardiac death.

▶ **What does the clinician want to know?**
Number, location, and degree of coronary stenoses • Signs of heart failure • LV enlargement • EF (important prognostic indicator!).

Differential Diagnosis

Coronary anomalies	– Anomalous origin of the coronary arteries
	– Life-threatening variant: ALCA, most symptomatic during exercise
Syndrome X	– Angina pectoris
	– Angiographically normal coronary arteries
Cardiomyopathies	– Impaired LV function
	– Angiographically normal coronary arteries

Tips and Pitfalls

Suspicion of CHD warrants early investigation of coronary status and individualized risk assessment to assess prognosis and provide optimum treatment.

Selected References

Raff GL et al. Diagnostic accuracy of noninvasive coronary angiography using 64-slice spiral computed tomography. J Am Coll Cardiol 2005; 46: 552–557

Sardanelli F et al. Three-dimensional, navigator-echo MR coronary angiography in detecting stenoses of the major epicardial vessels, with conventional coronary angiography as the standard of reference. Radiology 2000; 214: 808–814

Smith SC. Current and future directions of cardiovascular risk prediction. Am J Cardiol 2006; 97: 28A–32A

Definition

▶ **Epidemiology**
Same as CHD (see above) • In 15–25% of patients, myocardial infarction occurs during the first 3 months.

▶ **Definition**
Initial manifestation or acutely progressive angina pectoris (e.g., occurs at progressively lower stress levels with symptomatic interval > 15 min) • Distinguished from infarction without ST-segment elevation • Markedly increased risk of myocardial infarction.

▶ **Etiology, pathophysiology, pathogenesis**
Acute coronary insufficiency due to a high-grade or hemodynamically significant stenosis • Usually based on atherosclerotic wall changes in CHD.

Imaging Signs

▶ **Modality of choice**
Invasive coronary angiography.

▶ **Chest radiograph findings**
Usually normal • Important to exclude signs of heart failure (pulmonary venous congestion, pulmonary edema, enlarged cardiac silhouette, pleural effusion).

▶ **Echocardiographic findings**
Regional wall motion abnormalities of varying degrees • Diastolic dysfunction precedes systolic dysfunction.

▶ **Nuclear medicine and PET**
Not indicated.

▶ **CT findings**
Particularly useful for rapid exclusion of other diagnoses in patients with acute chest pain • Atherosclerosis of coronary arteries • Coronary stenosis (multidetector CT).

▶ **MRI findings**
Not indicated in clinically unstable patients • Pharmacologic stress testing is absolutely contraindicated.

▶ **Invasive diagnostic procedures**
Coronary angiography • PTCA • Possible stent implantation.

Clinical Aspects

▶ **Typical presentation**
Progression of severity • Increasing severity and duration of episodes (crescendo angina) • Possible angina at rest.

▶ **Treatment options**
Myocardial revascularization: PTCA • Stent implantation • Possible aortocoronary bypass (e.g., as an alternative treatment for **truncal stenosis of the LCA).**

▶ **Course and prognosis**
Acute risk of myocardial infarction (up to 25%).

Fig. 1.8 Unstable angina pectoris in a 64-year-old man. Coronary angiogram of the LCA shows multiple coronary stenoses (arrows) of varying degrees of severity including high-grade lesions.

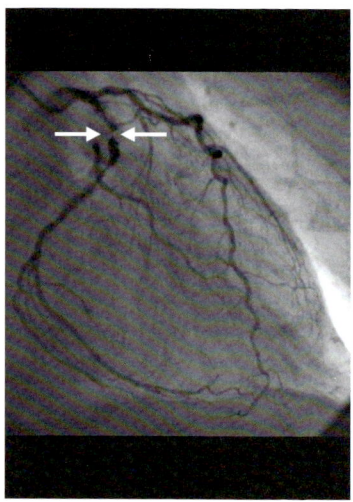

Fig. 1.9 Coronary angiogram in the same patient as in Fig. 1.8. Multiple LCA stenoses including high-grade lesions (arrows).

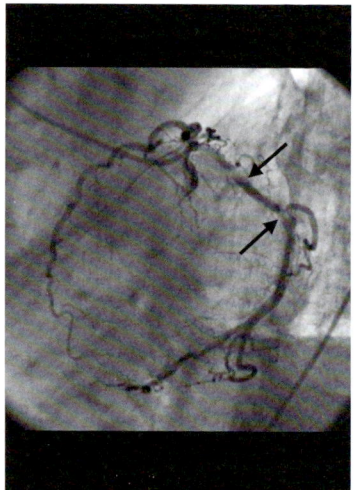

▶ **What does the clinician want to know?**

Atherosclerotic wall changes • Coronary stenosis (multidetector CT) • LV function, signs of decompensation.

Differential Diagnosis

Acute chest pain	– Acute myocardial infarction
	– Aortic dissection
	– Pulmonary embolism
	– Myocarditis
Other coronary diseases	– Coronary dissection
	– Coronary anomalies
	– Prinzmetal angina

Tips and Pitfalls

Unstable angina pectoris, like acute myocardial infarction, should be recognized as an emergency that warrants immediate treatment.

Selected References

Spaulding C et al. Management of acute coronary syndromes. N Engl J Med 2005; 353: 2714–2718

Yan RT et al. Canadian Acute Coronary Syndromes (ACS) Registry Investigators. Age-related differences in the management and outcome of patients with acute coronary syndromes. Am Heart J 2006; 151: 352–359

Definition

▶ **Epidemiology**
Leading cause of death in Western countries • Prevalence approximately 2.5% • Outcome is fatal in 30% • More than half of all deaths occur in prehospital settings.

▶ **Etiology, pathophysiology, pathogenesis**
Approximately 95% of all AMIs result from atherosclerotic lesions of the coronary arteries • All cases are caused by an acute coronary artery occlusion that critically restricts blood flow to the myocardium • Necrosis of myocardial tissue • *ECG:* ST-segment elevation infarction.

Imaging Signs

▶ **Modality of choice**
Conventional coronary angiography.

▶ **Chest radiograph findings**
Often normal • Severe infarction leads to cardiac decompensation and imaging signs of heart failure • Pulmonary venous congestion • Pulmonary edema • Pleural effusion • Enlarged cardiac silhouette.

▶ **Echocardiography**
Impaired ventricular function • Regional wall motion abnormalities of varying degrees • Acute mitral insufficiency is seen with papillary muscle rupture • Detection of intracavitary thrombus.

▶ **CT findings**
Useful for rapid exclusion of other diagnoses in patients with acute chest pain • Atherosclerosis of coronary arteries • Coronary stenosis (multidetector CT) • May show decreased perfusion in the infarcted myocardial segment • May demonstrate a thrombus.

▶ **MRI findings**
Functional findings same as echocardiography • Perfusion defect • Increased T2-weighted signal intensity (edema) and delayed contrast enhancement of the infarcted area • Thrombus detection • Usually not indicated during the first 24 hours.

▶ **Invasive diagnostic procedures**
Coronary angiography • PTCA • Possible stent implantation • Regional and/or global LV dysfunction.

Clinical Aspects

▶ **Typical presentation**
Extremely severe ("crushing") precordial pain of acute onset • Cold sweats • Signs of acute heart failure • Arrhythmia • 15–20% of patients do not experience chest pain ("silent heart attack").

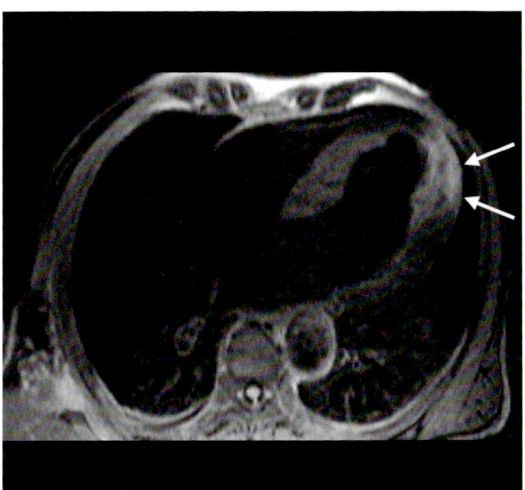

Fig. 1.10 Antero-lateral myocardial infarction in a 68-year-old man. Dark-blood T2-weighted TSE sequence (four-chamber view) shows hyperintense signal intensity due to myocardial edema in the infarcted area (arrow).

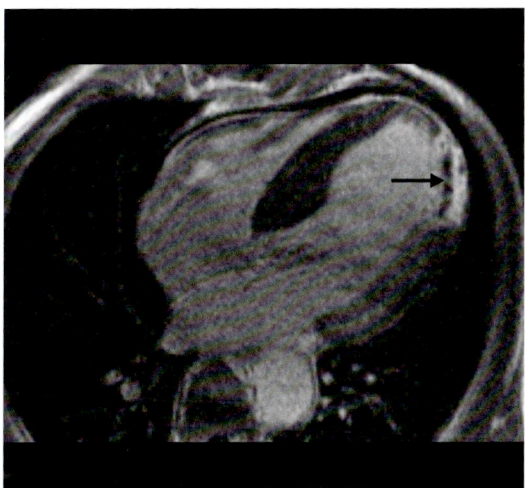

Fig. 1.11 Imaging with i.v. administration of gadolinium-DTPA. The hyperintense infarcted area shows delayed contrast enhancement with a central non-enhancing zone of low signal intensity (arrow, "no reflow" phenomenon).

▶ **Treatment options**
Acute therapy: Oxygen, morphine, platelet aggregation inhibitors, nitrates, β-blockers, acute PTCA (treatment of choice) • Systemic thrombolysis for ischemia of < 3 hours' duration.

▶ **Course and prognosis**
Sixty percent of deaths from AMI occur during the first 60 minutes.

▶ **What does the clinician want to know?**
Signs of heart failure such as pulmonary venous congestion • Pulmonary edema • Pleural effusion • Infarcted area (CT, MRI) • Coronary occlusion.

Differential Diagnosis

Acute chest pain	– Pulmonary embolism
	– Aortic dissection
	– Peri- or myocarditis, apical ballooning
Other coronary diseases	– Coronary anomalies
	– Prinzmetal angina

Tips and Pitfalls

Always consider AMI in the differential diagnosis of patients with acute chest pain, even when the clinical presentation is relatively unimpressive.

Selected References

Antman EM et al. ACC/AHA guidelines for the management of patients with ST-elevation myocardial infarction. Circulation 2004; 110: e82–292

Braunwald E et al. ACC/AHA 2002 guideline update for the management of patients with unstable angina and non-ST-segment elevation myocardial infarction—summary article: a report of the American College of Cardiology/American Heart Association task force on practice guidelines (Committee on the Management of Patients With Unstable Angina). J Am Coll Cardiol 2002; 40: 1366–1374

Edelman RR. Contrast-enhanced MR Imaging of the Heart: Overview of the Literature. Radiology 2004; 232: 653–668

Definition

▶ **Epidemiology**
Approximately 70% of myocardial infarctions advance to a chronic stage.
▶ **Pathoanatomy, classification**
History of an ischemic event at least 3 months earlier.
▶ **Etiology, pathophysiology, pathogenesis**
Follows acute myocardial infarction ● Regional myocardial necrosis, which is replaced by fibrotic scar tissue ● Rarely, the infarcted area may undergo calcification or fatty dystrophy.

Imaging Signs

▶ **Modality of choice**
Echocardiography.
▶ **Chest radiograph findings**
Often normal in patients with compensated heart function ● May show enlargement of the cardiac silhouette ● Chronic pulmonary venous congestion ● Congestive pulmonary fibrosis due to recurrent decompensation.
▶ **Echocardiographic findings**
Decreased regional wall thickness ● Functional impairment ranging from mild hypokinesia to dyskinesia ● LV dilatation.
▶ **Nuclear medicine and PET findings**
Reduced tracer uptake in the scar ● Detection and quantification of myocardial dysfunction.
▶ **CT findings**
Decreased wall thickness in the scarred area ● Possible perfusion defect.
▶ **MRI findings**
Findings same as echocardiography and CT ● Decreased myocardial perfusion and delayed contrast enhancement of the myocardial scar after administration of gadolinium-DTPA.
▶ **Invasive diagnostic procedures**
Coronary angiography: Regional and/or global LV dysfunction ● Possible PTCA or stent implantation.

Clinical Aspects

▶ **Typical presentation**
Heart failure with possible dyspnea on exertion or at rest ● Possible pulmonary edema ● Signs of superior and/or inferior vena cava obstruction ● Arrhythmias.
▶ **Treatment options**
Stabilization of heart failure with medical treatment ● Stent implantation or aortocoronary bypass in patients with angina pectoris or progressive heart failure ● Secondary prevention.

Fig. 1.12 Chronic myocardial infarction. P-A chest radiograph shows cardiomegaly in association with decompensated left heart failure, LV dilatation, and chronic pulmonary venous congestion.

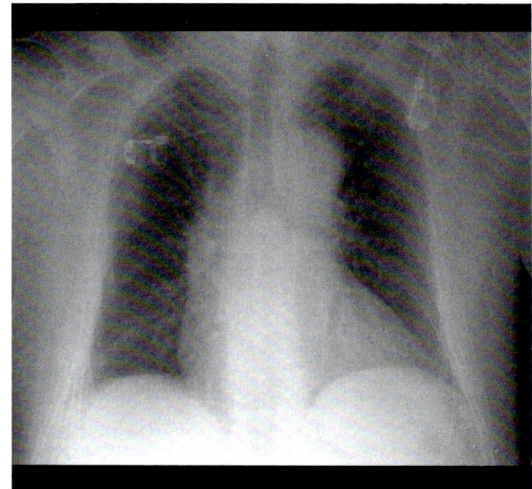

Fig. 1.13 Same patient as in Fig. 1.**12**. MR image (IR GE sequence, short-axis view) acquired 15 minutes after gadolinium-DTPA administration shows a hyperintense scar (delayed enhancement, arrows).

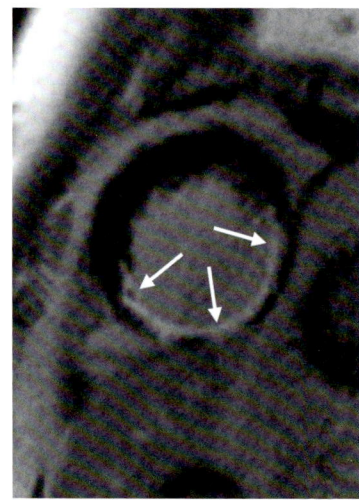

▶ **Course and prognosis**

Highly variable • Depend on the location, number, and degree of severity of stenotic lesions, LV function, and the progression of coronary sclerosis.

▶ **What does the clinician want to know?**

Ventricular function • Signs of heart failure • Myocardial viability • Secondary complications (ventricular aneurysm, ventricular thrombus).

Differential Diagnosis

Other causes of heart failure   – Cardiomyopathy
                                             – Chronic lung disease
                                             – Cardiac arrhythmia

Tips and Pitfalls

An unknown proportion of unrecognized ("silent") myocardial infarctions are prognostically important with abnormalities detectable on multidetector CT and MRI.

Selected References

Parisi AF. Clinical trials of coronary revascularization for chronic stable angina: medical treatment versus coronary revascularization. Curr Opin Cardiol 2000; 15: 275–280

Wu E et al. Visualisation of presence, location, and transmural extent of healed Q-wave and non-Q-wave myocardial infarction. Lancet 2001; 357: 21–28

Definition

▶ **Epidemiology**
Complicates up to 10% of myocardial infarctions with ST-segment elevation.
▶ **Pathoanatomy, classification**
Aneurysmal dilatation of a myocardial region ● Most commonly develops at the LV apex ● Occasionally forms on the lateral or inferior LV wall or in the RV.
▶ **Etiology, pathophysiology, pathogenesis**
Usually results from an extensive transmural myocardial infarction ● Other causes (myocarditis, ARVC, trauma, postoperative) ● Decreased wall elasticity due to structural myocardial changes (scar tissue, fatty dysplasia) ● This leads to dilatation in response to physiologic pressures ● Impaired cardiac output due to dead-space volume.

Imaging Signs

▶ **Modality of choice**
Echocardiography.
▶ **Chest radiograph findings**
LV dilatation or cardiomegaly ● Possible signs of chronic congestion.
▶ **Echocardiographic findings**
Ventricular dilatation ● Dyskinesia of the aneurysm ● Global functional impairment (EF < 50%) ● Possible thrombi.
▶ **CT findings**
Dilated ventricle with an aneurysm ● Thrombus detection.
▶ **MRI findings**
Same findings as echocardiography and CT ● Delayed enhancement after gadolinium administration of postinfarction scar ● Other structural myocardial changes (e.g., T1-weighted TSE if ARVC is suspected).
▶ **Invasive diagnostic procedures**
Left ventriculography: Dilated ventricle with an aneurysm and dyskinesia ● Coronary stenosis in patients with CHD ● Echocardiography, CT, and MRI are superior for thrombus detection.

Clinical Aspects

▶ **Typical presentation**
Signs of heart failure ● Possible features of CHD with angina pectoris, dyspnea, and cardiac arrhythmias ● Possible recurrent emboli (cerebral ischemic attacks, "cold leg," etc.).
▶ **Treatment options**
Anticoagulant medication ● Large aneurysms that significantly compromise ventricular function may require surgical aneurysmectomy ● Cardiac pacemaker.
▶ **Course and prognosis**
Mortality depends on aneurysm size, ventricular function, and the time since the myocardial infarction (early onset after AMI is a poor prognostic sign).

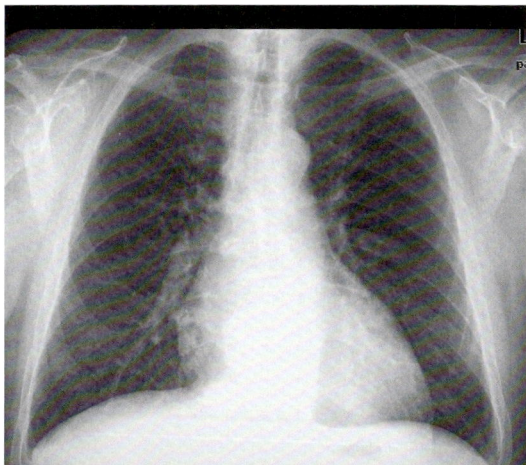

Fig. 1.14 A 56-year-old man who sustained a myocardial infarction 4 years earlier. P-A chest radiograph shows LV dilatation and chronic pulmonary venous congestion. Echocardiography documented severe impairment of LV function (EF 37%).

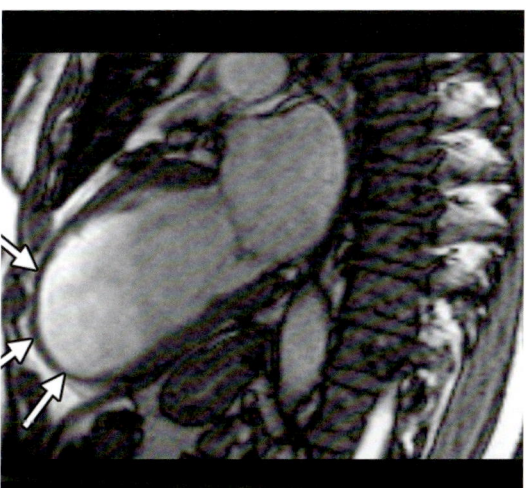

Fig. 1.15 SSFP sequence in the same patient as in Fig. 1.14. Long-axis view parallel to the septum shows a markedly enlarged LV with an apical aneurysm (arrows) in the infarcted area.

Fig. 1.16 Same patient as in Figs 1.**14** and 1.**15**. SSFP image, four-chamber view, showing extensive apical aneurysm and secondary tricuspid insufficiency in the setting of chronic LV decompensation and right-heart overload (arrow). Bilateral pleural effusions (*) are also present.

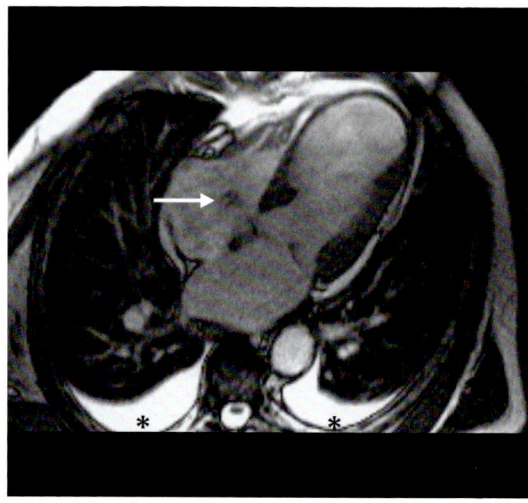

▶ **What does the clinician want to know?**

Size and location of the aneurysm • Ventricular thrombus • Ventricular function (EF) • Signs of heart failure.

Differential Diagnosis

Cardiomyopathy	– Global ventricular dilatation in DCM
Coronary heart disease	– Pseudoaneurysm due to acute infarction and myocardial perforation (caution: pericardial tamponade)
Other causes	– Intra- and extrapericardial masses (malignant tumor, cyst) and thoracic malformations can mimic a ventricular aneurysm on chest radiographs (should be supplemented with sectional imaging).

Tips and Pitfalls

Ventricular aneurysms are prone to thrombus formation and arterial emboli • Therefore a thrombus should be excluded.

Selected References

Heatlie GJ et al. Left ventricular aneurysm: comprehensive assessment of morphology, structure and thrombus using cardiovascular magnetic resonance. Clin Radiol 2005; 60: 687–692

Yeo TC et al. Clinical profile and outcome in 52 patients with cardiac pseudoaneurysm. Ann Intern Med 1998; 128: 299–305

Definition

▶ **Epidemiology**
Cardiac syndrome X is believed to occur in some patients with angina pectoris and a normal coronary angiogram • It should not be confused with metabolic syndrome X (obesity, hyperlipidemia, insulin resistance, hyperinsulinemia, and arterial hypertension).

▶ **Etiology, pathophysiology, pathogenesis**
Presumably based on microvascular coronary disease with endothelial dysfunction • No morphologic changes seen in the large coronary arteries • Stress-induced angina pectoris.

Imaging Signs

▶ **Modality of choice**
Coronary angiography.

▶ **Chest radiograph findings**
No cardiopulmonary abnormalities.

▶ **Echocardiographic findings**
Normal ventricular function at rest • Possible dysfunction during stress.

▶ **SPECT, PET, and MRI findings**
Decreased subendocardial perfusion reserve and perfusion defect during stress (adenosine) • No infarcted area which otherwise would present as a fixed defect of tracer uptake (nuclear medicine) or region of delayed contrast enhancement (MRI).

▶ **CT and invasive diagnostic procedures**
Multidetector CT or coronary angiography to exclude stenosis of major coronary vessels.

Clinical Aspects

▶ **Typical presentation**
Typical clinical presentation of angina pectoris (retrosternal pain, tightness in the chest, exertional dyspnea) • Abnormal stress ECG.

▶ **Treatment options**
Antianginal medication • Reduction of atherogenic risk factors.

▶ **Course and prognosis**
No effect on survival rate • Impaired quality of life.

▶ **What does the clinician want to know?**
Exclusion of CHD and its sequelae such as left-sided heart failure, ventricular dysfunction, and myocardial infarction.

Fig. 1.17 Cardiac syndrome X in a 54-year-old man. Adenosine stress perfusion MR image shows a circumferential, subendocardial perfusion deficit consistent with impaired microcirculation (arrows). Coronary angiograms were normal in this case.

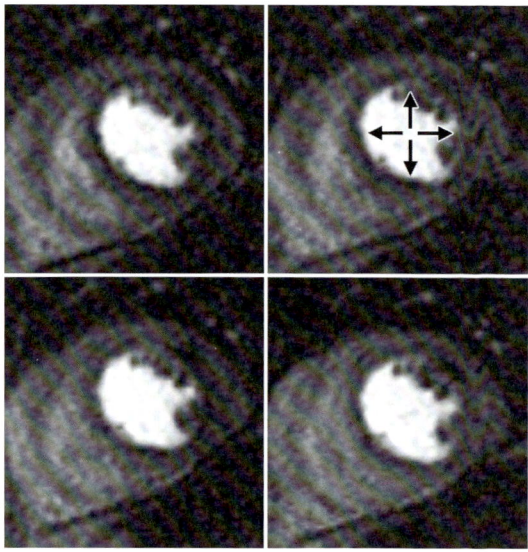

Differential Diagnosis

Cardiac causes	– CHD
	– Prinzmetal angina
	– Coronary anomaly
Other causes	– Dysphagia
	– Reflux disease

Tips and Pitfalls

Other causes should be investigated in patients with typical clinical features of stress-induced angina pectoris and normal coronary arteries.

Selected References

Panting JR et al. Abnormal subendocardial perfusion in cardiac syndrome X detected by cardiovascular magnetic resonance imaging. N Engl J Med 2002; 346: 1948–1953

Pasqui AL et al. Structural and functional abnormality of systemic microvessels in cardiac syndrome X. Nutr Metab Cardiovasc Dis 2005; 15: 56–64

Definition

▶ **Epidemiology**
Rarest form of angina pectoris • Most common between 20 and 40 years of age.

▶ **Etiology, pathophysiology, pathogenesis**
Special form of angina pectoris • Reversible ST-segment elevation • No rise in enzyme levels • Caused by coronary artery vasospasm or relatively high-grade atherosclerotic wall changes.

Imaging Signs

▶ **Modality of choice**
ECG and invasive coronary angiography, supported if necessary by provocative drug testing.

▶ **Chest radiograph findings**
No cardiopulmonary abnormalities.

▶ **Echocardiographic findings**
May demonstrate regional wall motion abnormalities (hypo- or akinesia) in acute ischemia.

▶ **Invasive diagnostic procedures**
Acute coronary artery spasm on coronary angiography in response to provocative testing.

Clinical Aspects

▶ **Typical presentation**
Angina pectoris • Symptoms are usually present at rest, rarely stress induced • Often present during morning hours.

▶ **Treatment options**
Pharmacologic therapy (nitrates) • May need to eliminate precipitating physical exertion.

▶ **Course and prognosis**
Variable • Dangerous cardiac arrhythmias may occur during an episode • Possible myocardial infarction or heart failure.

▶ **What does the clinician want to know?**
Exclusion of CHD and other possible causes in patients with acute chest pain.

Differential Diagnosis

Acute chest pain	– Acute coronary syndrome
	– Syndrome X
	– Coronary anomaly
	– Aortic dissection
	– Pulmonary embolism

Tips and Pitfalls

History points to the correct diagnosis • Prinzmetal angina should be included in the differential diagnosis of patients with suggestive symptoms and angiographically normal coronary arteries.

Selected References

Holt DB et al. Images in cardiovascular medicine. Prinzmetal angina in an adolescent: adjunctive role of tissue synchronization imaging. Circulation 2005; 112: 91–92

Keller KB, Lemberg L. Prinzmetal's angina. Am J Crit Care 2004; 13: 350–354

Definition

▶ **Epidemiology**
Aortocoronary bypass has been a routine myocardial revascularization procedure for the past 30 years • Involves the placement of arteriovenous bypass grafts.

▶ **Pathoanatomy, classification**
The bypass vessel is anastomosed distal to the stenotic vascular segment • Several types are distinguished:
– Arterial bypass (e.g., internal thoracic artery).
– Venous bypass (e.g., long saphenous vein).
– Monograft bypass (bypassing one coronary artery with one anastomosis).
– Sequential bypass (bypassing multiple coronary arteries with several consecutive anastomoses).

▶ **Etiology, pathophysiology, pathogenesis**
Atherosclerotic wall changes in the coronary arteries lead to myocardial ischemia • Principal indications for aortocoronary bypass grafting are **main-trunk disease and failed PTCA.**

Imaging Signs

▶ **Modality of choice**
Invasive coronary angiography.

▶ **Chest radiograph findings**
May show signs of chronic left heart overload • Mediastinal clip material (thoracic arterial graft) • Sternal cerclage wires.

▶ **Echocardiographic findings**
Regional dysfunction • Possible myocardial scar • Occasional akinesia or dyskinesia of myocardial regions • Possible impairment of LV function.

▶ **CT findings**
CT angiography can demonstrate coronary arteries and bypass grafts • Detection of bypass occlusion or stenosis • May be of limited value in evaluating the anastomoses • Only multidetector CT (16 rows or more) should be used.

▶ **MRI findings**
Functional findings same as echocardiography • Delayed contrast enhancement of myocardial scar • MR angiography of bypass grafts • Flow can be quantified and the flow reserve determined by phase-contrast velocity mapping.

▶ **Invasive diagnostic procedures**
Coronary angiography with selective visualization of the bypass vessels and coronary arteries • Visualization of vascular stenoses and occlusions • Left ventriculogram with assessment of myocardial function.

Fig. 1.18 Aorto-coronary bypass surgery. P-A chest radiograph shows an enlarged LV with no signs of acute congestion. There is mild chronic pulmonary venous congestion with increased perfusion of the upper lobe vessels. Cerclage wires from a previous sternotomy are also visible.

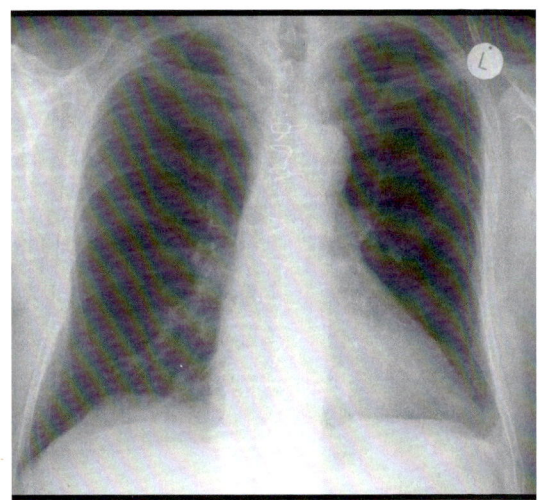

Fig. 1.19a, b Multidetector CT (**a**) and coronary angiogram (**b**) following aortocoronary bypass grafting (venous bypass to the LAD). The anastomotic site (arrow) appears normal.

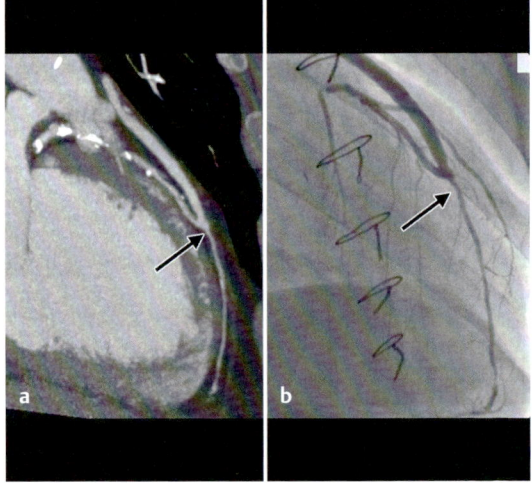

Clinical Aspects

▶ **Typical presentation**
No clinical complaints following successful myocardial revascularization • Recurrence of angina pectoris suggests restenosis of the coronary arteries or bypass grafts.

▶ **Treatment options**
PTCA and stent implantation for coronary or bypass stenosis • Possible need for reoperation (aortocoronary bypass) • Medical treatment following the therapeutic guidelines for CHD.

▶ **Course and prognosis**
Average operative risk is 3% • EF < 35% correlates with increased perioperative mortality • Prognosis depends on the surgical outcome and progression of underlying disease (CHD) • *Signs of poor prognosis:* Heart failure, angina pectoris, diabetes mellitus, acute myocardial infarction, chronic obstructive lung disease • Up to 90% 5-year survival rate, 80% 10-year survival rate.

▶ **What does the clinician want to know?**
Regional and global ventricular function • Postinfarction scar • Bypass patency • Evaluation of anastomosis • LV dilatation • Signs of decompensation.

Differential Diagnosis

Progression of CHD	– Angina pectoris
Sternal nonunion after sternotomy	– Chest pain
Cardiomyopathy (e.g., DCM)	– Left-sided heart failure

Selected References

Salm LP et al. Functional significance of stenoses in coronary artery bypass grafts. Evaluation by single-photon emission computed tomography perfusion imaging, cardiovascular magnetic resonance, and angiography. J Am Coll Cardiol 2004; 44: 1877–1882

Schoepf UJ et al. CT of coronary artery disease. Radiology 2004; 232: 18–37

Definition

▶ **Synonyms**
ALCA (anomalous origin of the LCA) • ARCA (anomalous origin of the RCA).
▶ **Epidemiology**
Frequently associated with other congenital malformations of the heart • Noted in up to 6% of patients undergoing cardiac CT scans.
▶ **Pathoanatomy, classification**
ALCA: Ectopic origin of the LCA or its branches (LAD, RCX) from the right sinus of Valsalva.
ARCA: Ectopic origin of the RCA from the left sinus of Valsalva.
▶ **Etiology, pathophysiology, pathogenesis**
Congenital malformation of unknown etiology • The interarterial course of the main trunk of the LCA between the roots of the aorta and pulmonary artery is clinically important ("malignant" variant of ALCA, approximately 10% of all congenital coronary anomalies; see p. 294).

Imaging Signs

▶ **Modality of choice**
Multidetector CT or MRI.
▶ **Chest radiograph findings**
No cardiopulmonary abnormalities.
▶ **Echocardiographic findings**
TTE or TEE: Anomalous origin from the aortic root.
▶ **CT and MRI findings**
These studies supplement echocardiographic findings by defining the precise course of the vessels • May demonstrate kinking, compression, or entrapment (malignant variant of ALCA).
▶ **Invasive diagnostic procedures**
Coronary angiography demonstrates the anomalous origin of the LCA or ALCA • May demonstrate stenoses and collaterals.

Clinical Aspects

▶ **Typical presentation**
Clinical hallmarks are exercise-induced syncope, atrial fibrillation, transient LBBB, chest pain, and anxiety.
▶ **Treatment options**
The preferred treatment in symptomatic patients is corrective surgical reimplantation of the aberrant coronary artery • Another option is bypass grafting.
▶ **Course and prognosis**
The benign, asymptomatic variant has a good prognosis • There is up to a 50% risk of life-threatening stress-induced complications in the malignant variant of ALCA.

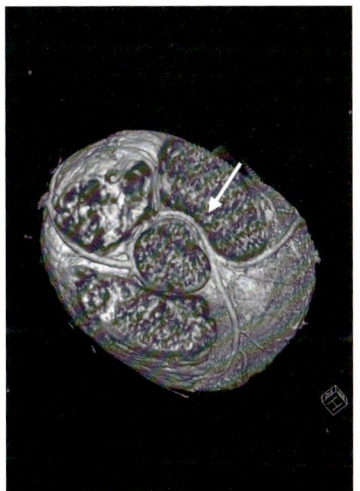

Fig. 1.20 ECG-triggered MDCT in a 26-year-old man who experienced syncope during athletic activity. Contrast-enhanced SSD demonstrates anomalous origin of the LCA (ALCA, arrow).

▶ **What does the clinician want to know?**
Origin and course of the aberrant coronary arteries, stenosis, collaterals, and myocardial function.

Differential Diagnosis

Coronary fistulae with anomalous termination (80% right cardiac, 10% left cardiac, 10% other; RCA affected in 60% of cases, LCA in 30%), CHD, coronary dissection, vasculitis.

Tips and Pitfalls

Coronary anomalies are an important differential diagnosis in younger patients without cardiac symptoms ● Hence it is important to evaluate the aortic root and the origins of the coronary arteries with echocardiography, CT, or MRI.

Selected References

Angelini P. Normal and anomalous coronary arteries: definitions and classification. Am Heart J 1989; 117: 418–434

Datta J et al. Anomalous Coronary Arteries in Adults: Depiction at Multi–Detector Row CT Angiography. Radiology 2005; 235: 812–818

Definition

▶ **Epidemiology**
Most important symptomatic coronary arterial anomaly in children • Present in 1:3000 newborns • *Synonym:* ALCAPA (anomalous origin of the LCA from the pulmonary artery).

▶ **Etiology, pathophysiology, pathogenesis**
Anomalous origin of the LCA from the left pulmonary artery • Harmless before birth because the pulmonary and systemic circulations have similar oxygen saturation and pressure levels • When the pressures change after birth the blood and oxygen supply to the LV is insufficient • Without collateral flow from the RCA, myocardial infarction may occur.

Imaging Signs

▶ **Modality of choice**
Coronary angiography.

▶ **Chest radiograph findings**
Often normal • May show LV dilatation with signs of ischemia and heart failure.

▶ **Echocardiography findings**
LV dilatation and dysfunction • Collateral vessels.

▶ **Nuclear medicine findings**
Large perfusion defect in the LV.

▶ **CT findings**
Anomalous origin of the LCA from the left pulmonary artery • LV dilatation.

▶ **MRI findings**
Same findings as echocardiography and CT • Myocardial perfusion and viability can also be evaluated on gadolinium-enhanced images (delayed contrast enhancement) • Flow measurement in the LCA.

▶ **Invasive diagnostic procedures**
Define the origin of the LCA from the left pulmonary artery • Define collateral vessels arising from the RCA • Retrograde perfusion of the LCA.

Clinical Aspects

▶ **Typical presentation**
Symptoms usually appear during the first weeks of life • Failure to thrive • Heart failure • Mitral insufficiency • Myocardial ischemia • Possible myocardial infarction • Approximately 5–10% of cases do not become symptomatic until adulthood.

▶ **Treatment options**
Symptomatic patients require immediate treatment for heart failure and prompt surgical intervention (emergency indication) • Treatment of choice is reimplantation of the LCA into the aorta • Coronary bypass surgery is rarely necessary.

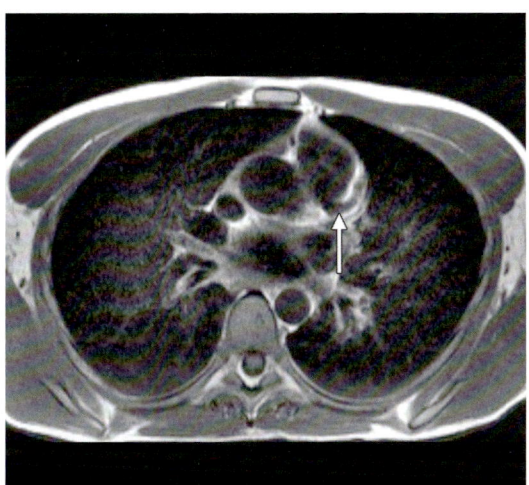

Fig. 1.21 A 26-year-old man with Bland–White–Garland syndrome. Axial, T1-weighted MR image (TSE sequence) showing the LCA arising from the pulmonary trunk (arrow).

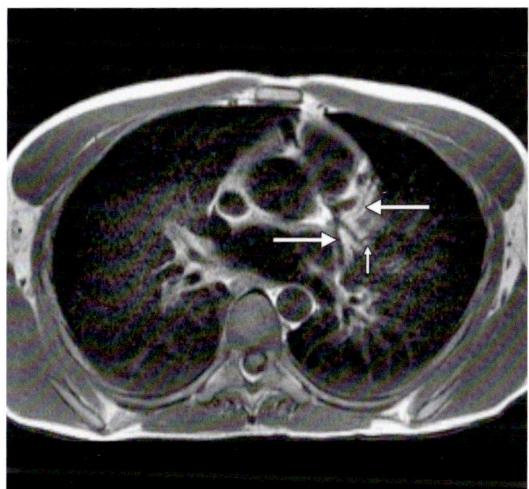

Fig. 1.22 The next lower slice in the same patient as in Fig. 1.**21** shows the division of the LCA into the LAD, LCX, and an intermediate branch (arrows).

Fig. 1.23 Magnified view of Fig. 1.**22** showing the LAD, LCX, and an intermediate branch (arrows).

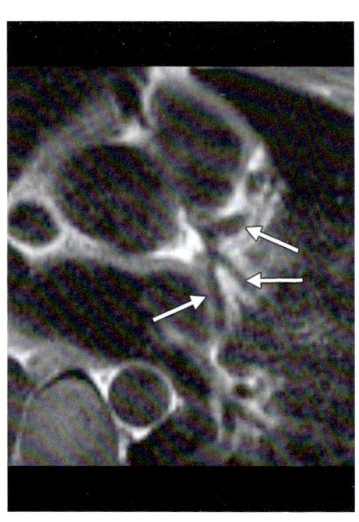

▶ **Course and prognosis**

Normal LV function is reestablished soon after surgery • The risk of sudden cardiac death is minimized • Good prognosis after successful operative treatment.

▶ **What does the clinician want to know?**

Origin of the LCA • Collaterals from the RCA • Myocardial viability • Mitral insufficiency.

Differential Diagnosis

Other coronary anomalies – E.g., ALCA, ARCA

Tips and Pitfalls

Bland–White–Garland syndrome requires differentiation from CHD, especially in younger adults • *Caution:* High risk associated with stress testing (e.g. adenosine infusion).

Selected References

Bruder O et al. Magnetic resonance imaging of anomalous origin of the left coronary artery from the pulmonary artery (Bland-White-Garland syndrome). Heart 2005; 91: 656

Cowie MR et al. The diagnosis and assessment of an adult with anomalous origin of the left coronary artery from the pulmonary artery. Eur J Nucl Med 1994; 21: 1017–1019

Definition

▶ **Epidemiology**
Rare in Europe and the U.S.A. • Predominantly affects children under 5 years of age • Most common vasculitis in small children • Involves the coronary vessels in approximately 25% of cases.

▶ **Etiology, pathophysiology, pathogenesis**
Vasculitis of unknown cause • Presumably has an infectious etiology in which superantigens (bacteria-produced toxins) have a role.
Stages:
– Acute febrile phase (up to 2 weeks).
– Subacute phase (up to 6 weeks).
– Convalescent phase (6–8 weeks).

Imaging Signs

▶ **Modality of choice**
Echocardiography.

▶ **Chest radiograph findings**
Radiographic findings range from normal to cardiomegaly or pulmonary infiltrates depending on the severity.

▶ **Echocardiography findings**
Pericardial effusion • Valvular insufficiency • Myocardial dysfunction • Coronary aneurysms starting on about day 10 of the febrile phase.

▶ **CT and MRI findings**
Same as echocardiography findings • Multidetector CT angiography or MR angiography can detect aneurysms and evaluate the vessel wall • Aneurysms may exhibit partial thrombosis.

▶ **Invasive diagnostic procedures**
Coronary angiography shows irregular aneurysmal dilatations of the coronary arteries.

Clinical Aspects

▶ **Typical presentation**
Characteristic stages • Initial high fever that lasts 5–10 days and is unresponsive to antibiotics • Bilateral conjunctivitis • Enlarged cervical lymph nodes • Macular erythema on the palms • Approximately 25% of cases show cardiac involvement with development of coronary aneurysms.

▶ **Treatment options**
Investigate coronary status • Aneurysms require long-term aspirin and immunoglobulin therapy.

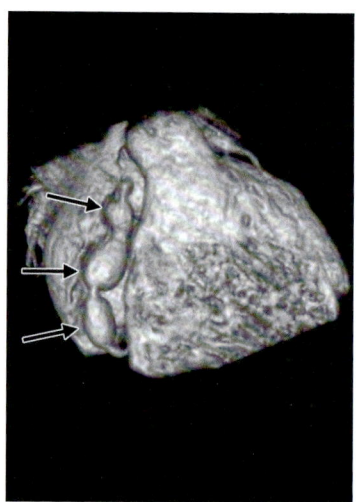

Fig. 1.24 Kawasaki syndrome in a 3-year-old child with coronary aneurysms. Three-dimensional surface reconstruction of an SSFP MR angiogram shows a series of aneurysms distributed along the RCA (arrows).

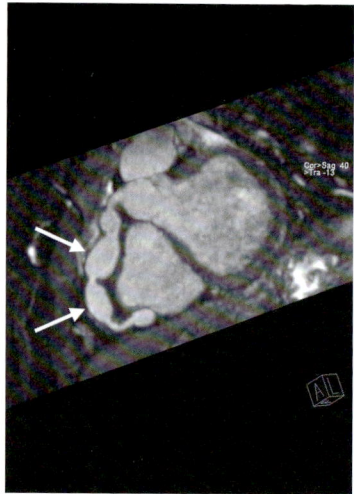

Fig. 1.25 Same patient as in Fig. 1.**24**. Curved MPR along the course of the RCA demonstrates multiple coronary aneurysms (arrows).

▶ **Course and prognosis**

Prompt diagnosis and early initiation of treatment will significantly influence prognosis • Approximately 50% of coronary aneurysms will regress within 1 year (risk levels I and II) • Persistent coronary stenoses • (Giant) aneurysms develop in 20% (risk levels III and IV) • Up to a third of patients will have a myocardial infarction during the first 3 years.

▶ **What does the clinician want to know?**

Aneurysms of the coronary arteries • Partial thrombosis (risk factor!) • Myocardial and cardiac valve function • Signs of myocardial infarction.

Differential Diagnosis

Coronary anomalies	– ALCA, ARCA (ectopic origin of the left or right coronary artery)

Tips and Pitfalls

Kawasaki syndrome should be considered in children under 5 years of age with persistent fever • Investigate by early echocardiography • Schedule echocardiographic or MRI follow-ups.

Selected References

Benseler SM etal. Infections and Kawasaki disease: implications for coronary artery outcome. Pediatrics. 2005; 116: e760–766

McMahon CJ et al. Detection of active coronary arterial vasculitis using magnetic resonance imaging in Kawasaki disease. Circulation 2005; 112: e315–e316

Definition

▶ **Classification**
Acute heart failure is classified into three categories:
– Acute decompensation of chronic heart failure.
– Acute cardiogenic pulmonary edema (rise in pulmonary capillary filling pressures).
– Cardiogenic shock (decreased cardiac output with arterial hypertension and decreased systemic blood flow).

▶ **Etiology, pathophysiology, pathogenesis**
Acute heart failure: Occurs in almost all diseases that lead to chronic heart failure ● Treatment noncompliance or pharmacologic side effects ● Renal failure ● Hyperthyroidism ● Infections.
Cardiogenic shock: Most common cause is acute myocardial infarction ● Aortic dissection ● Pericardial tamponade ● Cardiac trauma ● Pulmonary embolism ● Florid endocarditis with valvular dysfunction ● Postoperative myocardial dysfunction ● Myocardial depression in other forms of shock (e.g., septic shock).

▶ **Pathoanatomy**
Variable; depends on the underlying disease.

Imaging Signs

▶ **Modality of choice**
Echocardiography.

▶ **Chest radiograph findings**
Enlarged cardiac silhouette (may also be normal!) ● Increased pulmonary vascular markings with blood diversion to apical vessels ● Pulmonary edema ● Pleural effusion.

▶ **Echocardiographic findings**
Dilated cardiac chambers ● Hypertrophy ● Impaired ventricular function ● Possible valvular dysfunction ● Pericardial effusion ● Dilatation of the inferior vena cava.

▶ **CT findings**
Same as chest radiograph findings ● Possible evidence of underlying cause, such as pulmonary embolism, aortic dissection, or pneumonia.

▶ **Nuclear medicine, PET, and MRI**
Not indicated in acute situations.

▶ **Invasive diagnostic procedures**
Suspected acute coronary syndrome should be investigated by coronary angiography.

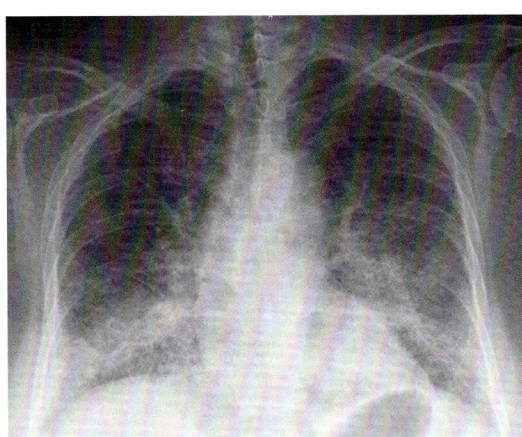

Fig. 2.1 Heart failure and alveolar pulmonary edema. Bedside A-P chest radiograph taken 4 hours after an acute myocardial infarction in a 69-year-old woman.

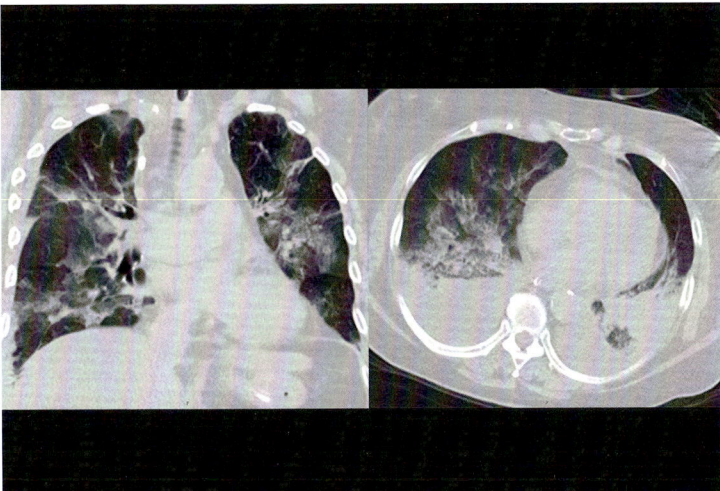

Fig. 2.2 Same patient as in Fig. 2.**1**. Unenhanced axial CT scan and reformatted coronal image show parahilar alveolar opacification due to pulmonary edema. Bilateral pleural effusions and basal dyselectasis are also present.

Clinical Aspects

▶ **Typical presentation**

Dyspnea ● Tachypnea ● Orthopnea ● Angina pectoris ● Tachycardia ● Distended neck veins ● Cold sweats ● Pallor ● Anxiety ● Restlessness.

▶ **Treatment options**

Treat the underlying disease whenever possible ● Oxygen ● Noninvasive ventilation or intubation, if required ● Morphine ● Reduce the afterload (e.g., with nitrates) if blood pressure is raised ● Patients with cardiogenic shock require careful treatment with catecholamines ● Revascularization ● Implantation of an intraaortic balloon pump.

▶ **Course and prognosis**

Mortality in cardiogenic shock is 50–70%.

▶ **What does the clinician want to know?**

Degree of severity ● Ventricular function ● Pulmonary edema ● Differentiation from pulmonary causes of dyspnea.

Differential Diagnosis

Other causes of dyspnea	– Restrictive or obstructive lung disease
	– Pneumonia
	– Pneumothorax
	– Pulmonary embolism
Other causes of shock	– Septic focus
	– Signs of hemorrhage (e.g., in whole-body CT)

Tips and Pitfalls

As acute heart failure has a wide-ranging differential diagnosis, the cause should always be thoroughly investigated.

Selected References

Antman EM et al. ACC/AHA guidelines for the management of patients with ST-elevation myocardial infarction. Circulation 2004; 110: 282–292

Kaul S. Doppler echocardiography in critically ill cardiac patients. Cardiol Clin 1991; 9: 711–732

Definition

▶ **Definition**
Systolic and/or diastolic abnormality of cardiac function in which the heart delivers insufficient oxygen to meet the body's needs.

▶ **Epidemiology, etiology**
One of the most common medical disorders ● Prevalence is 1.5–2% ● Prevalence increases with age, reaching 10% by 80 years ● Leading causes are CHD and arterial hypertension ● Cardiomyopathies ● Valvular heart disease ● Arrhythmias.

▶ **Pathoanatomy**
Variable; depends on the underlying disease.

Imaging Signs

▶ **Modality of choice**
Echocardiography.

▶ **Chest radiograph findings**
Enlargement of the cardiac silhouette (CTR > 2:1) ● Pulmonary venous congestion ● Kerley lines ● Pleural effusion.

▶ **Echocardiographic findings**
Dilatation of the atria and ventricles ● LV hypertrophy ● Scars and aneurysms ● Systolic and/or diastolic function impairment ● Valvular disease ● Pericardial effusion.

▶ **SPECT and PET findings**
Investigation of myocardial perfusion and viability.

▶ **CT findings**
Enlargement of the cardiac chambers ● Signs of congestion ● Pericardial and pleural effusion ● Pericardial, coronary, and valvular calcifications ● Evidence of CHD by multidetector CT angiography.

▶ **MRI findings**
Same as echocardiography and CT ● May show other signs of specific myocardial disease (sarcoidosis, hemochromatosis, amyloidosis, primary cardiomyopathies, myocarditis).

▶ **Invasive diagnostic procedures**
DD of CHD often requires coronary angiography ● Left ventriculography shows abnormal LV function and dilatation.

Clinical Aspects

▶ **Typical presentation**
Dyspnea ● Edema ● Fatigue ● Decreased exercise tolerance ● Gastrointestinal complaints ● Cardiac arrhythmias.

▶ **Treatment options**
Underlying disease is treated whenever possible ● Medical stabilization of heart failure ● Cardiac resynchronization if indicated ● ICD implantation or heart transplantation.

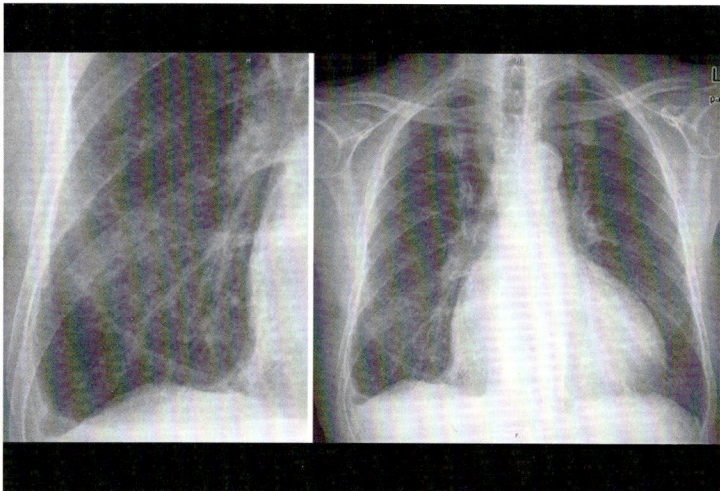

Fig. 2.3 Severe heart failure due to three-vessel CHD. Chest radiographs show cardio-megaly, pulmonary vascular dilatation, Kerley B lines, and an effusion in the right costo-phrenic angle.

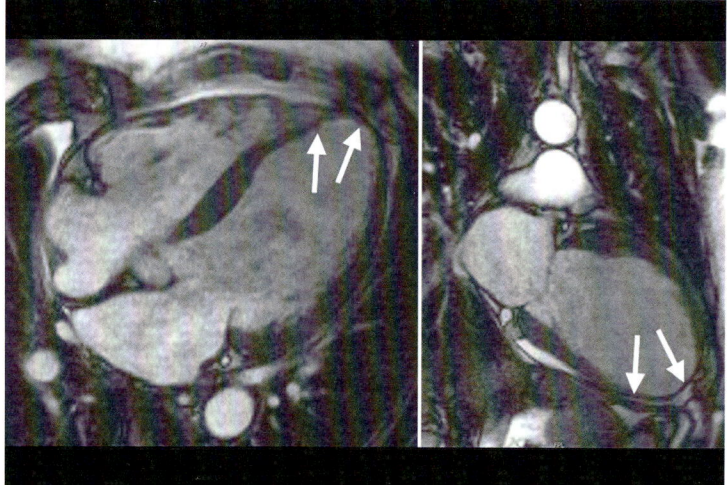

Fig. 2.4 MR image of the same patient as in Fig 2.**3**. SSFP images in the four-chamber and long-axis view demonstrate cardiomegaly along with apical and inferior postinfarc-tion scars (arrows).

▶ **Course and prognosis**
Usually progressive course • 2-year mortality of 40–50% in NYHA classes III and IV • Leading causes of death are cardiac failure and sudden cardiac death due to arrhythmia.

▶ **What does the clinician want to know?**
Morphologic and functional status of the heart • Signs indicating the etiology of the heart failure • Pulmonary signs of left-sided heart failure • Differentiation from pulmonary causes of dyspnea.

Differential Diagnosis

Other causes of dyspnea	– Restrictive or obstructive lung disease
	– Pneumonia
	– Chronic pulmonary embolism

Tips and Pitfalls

Findings in the chest radiograph correlate poorly with LV function • The findings should always be interpreted within the context of the clinical presentation and other imaging findings • MRI or CT of the heart often cannot be carried out in patients with atrial fibrillation or other tachycardias.

Selected References

Gerber BL et al. Accuracy of contrast-enhanced magnetic resonance imaging in predicting improvement of regional myocardial function in patients after acute myocardial infarction. Circulation 2002; 106: 1083–1089

Mangiavacchi M et al. Clinical predictors of marked improvement in left ventricular performance after cardiac resynchronization therapy in patients with chronic heart failure. Am Heart J 2006; 151: 477.e1–477.e6

Swedberg K et al. Guidelines for the diagnosis and treatment of chronic heart failure: executive summary (update 2005): The Task Force for the Diagnosis and Treatment of Chronic Heart Failure of the European Society of Cardiology. Eur Heart J 2005; 26: 1115–1140

Definition

▶ **Epidemiology, etiology**
Indications: Severe heart failure (NYHA class IV) with a life expectancy of less than 1 year • Leading reasons are CHD (45%) and dilated cardiomyopathy (45%).

▶ **Pathoanatomy, pathophysiology**
Same as for chronic heart failure prior to operation • Pathoanatomy is variable and depends on the etiology of acute heart failure.

Imaging Signs

▶ **Modality of choice**
Preoperative: Echocardiography • *Postoperative:* Echocardiography, myocardial biopsy if required.

▶ **Chest radiograph and CT findings**
Preoperative: Same as chronic heart failure.
Postoperative: Enlarged cardiac silhouette due to disproportion between donor heart and recipient pericardium • Pulmonary congestion or infection • Pneumomediastinum • Pneumothorax • Pneumopericardium and mediastinal widening • In some cases, pneumomediastinum and mediastinal widening may also be signs of mediastinitis (indication for CT).

▶ **Echocardiographic findings**
Preoperative: Same findings as in chronic heart failure • Cardiomegaly • Pericardial effusion • Abnormal ventricular function.
Postoperative: Acute rejection: myocardial wall thickening • Increased echogenicity • Pericardial effusion • Diastolic and systolic dysfunction.

▶ **CT findings**
Useful in long-term follow-up • Use of multidetector CT angiography to exclude allograft vasculopathy has not yet been evaluated but is plausible • In immunosuppressed patients to exclude secondary malignancies such as lymphoma, posttransplantation lymphoproliferative disorder (PTLD), skin tumors, visceral tumors, and Kaposi sarcoma.

▶ **MRI findings**
Preoperative: No routine indications.
Postoperative: Functional findings same as echocardiography • Rejection is marked by a focal or diffuse increase in T2 signal intensity • Increased myocardial enhancement after gadolinium-DTPA administration.

▶ **Invasive diagnostic procedures**
Preoperative (donor or recipient): Coronary angiography to exclude normal variants and CHD • *Postoperatively:* Right heart biopsy is the gold standard for confirming suspicion of acute rejection • In the long term, coronary angiography is the gold standard for the detection of allograft vasculopathy.

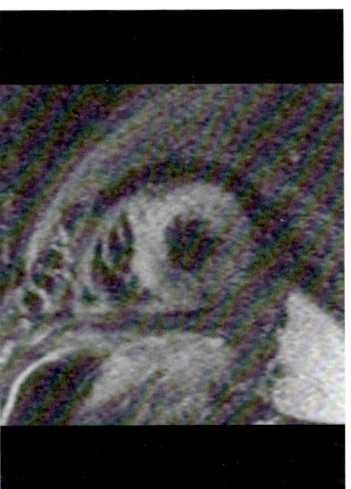

Fig. 2.5 Chronic rejection in a 63-year-old man in his fourth year after heart transplantation. Fat-saturated dark-blood T2-weighted TSE sequence, short-axis view shows marked myocardial hypertrophy and increased septal signal intensity due to chronic rejection.

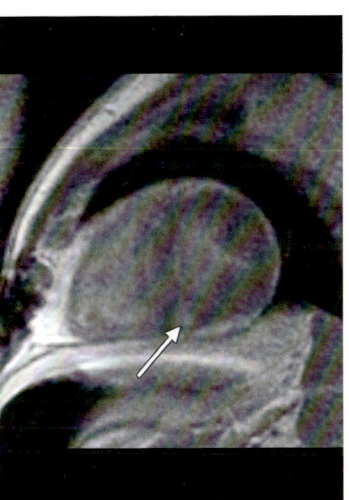

Fig. 2.6 Same patient as in Fig. 2.5. IR GE sequence after gadolinium administration shows diffuse enhancement with a relatively intense focus in the area of the inferior septum (arrow).

Clinical Aspects

▶ **Typical presentation**
Preoperative: Severe heart failure (NYHA class IV).
Postoperative: Same as in other cardiac surgery patients • Increased risk of infection due to immunosuppression.

▶ **Treatment options**

Treatment for heart failure • Immunosuppression • Treatment of infections • Secondary prophylaxis against CHD • Retransplantation.

▶ **Course and prognosis**

Acute rejection occurs in up to 55% of cases • Usually occurs between the second week and third month after heart transplantation • Mortality is highest during the first 6 months • 10-year survival rate up to 54% • Leading cause of death more than 1 year postoperatively is allograft vasculopathy (accelerated form of CHD, 50% prevalence at 5 years postoperatively) • Second leading cause of death is malignancy, especially lymphoproliferative disease.

▶ **What does the clinician want to know?**

Functional evaluation of the heart • Signs of rejection (MRI) • Postoperative complications • Infection • Malignant disease.

Differential Diagnosis

Postoperative mediastinal widening	– Normal postoperative finding
	– Mediastinitis
	– Mediastinal hemorrhage
	– Aortic dissection or pseudoaneurysm
Postoperative pulmonary infiltrates	– Bacterial pneumonia (e.g., Staphylococcal aureus, Pseudomonas, Klebsiella spp.)
	– Pulmonary aspergillosis
	– CMV pneumonia
	– Hemothorax

Tips and Pitfalls

Postoperative complications are often difficult to recognize on chest radiographs • Doubtful cases require prompt investigation by CT • Multidetector CT and MRI appear to be more important for long-term follow-up (currently under investigation) • MRI is strongly recommended whenever rejection is suspected.

Selected References

Bacal F et al. Normalization of right ventricular performance and remodeling evaluated by magnetic resonance imaging at late follow-up of heart transplantation: relationship between function, exercise capacity and pulmonary vascular resistance. J Heart Lung Transplant 2005; 24: 2031–2036

Chughtai A et al. Heart transplantation imaging in the adult. Semin Roentgenol. 2006; 41: 16–25

Chughtai A et al. Preoperative imaging in heart and lung transplantation in the adult. Semin Roentgenol 2006; 41: 26–35

Definition

▶ **Epidemiology**
Aortic stenosis may be congenital or acquired ● *Congenital aortic stenosis:* Approximately 5% of all cardiac anomalies ● Atherosclerotic changes are the most common cause of acquired aortic stenosis in patients over 70 years of age (prevalence of 3%).

▶ **Pathoanatomy, classification**
Narrowing of the valve orifice or LVOT.
Three types are distinguished:
– Valvular aortic stenosis (most common form).
– Supravalvular aortic stenosis (rare, congenital).
– Subvalvular aortic stenosis (e.g., in HOCM).
Grading of severity is based on the valve opening area (VOA):
– > 2 cm^2 Normal
– 1.5–2 cm^2 Mild
– 1.0–1.5 cm^2 Moderate
– < 1 cm^2 Severe
– < 0.7 cm^2 Critical

▶ **Etiology, pathophysiology, pathogenesis**
Degenerative changes are the most common cause of acquired aortic stenosis ● A bicuspid valve predisposes to aortic stenosis (approximately four times more common in males than females) and often becomes symptomatic at 40–60 years of age ● Rare cases are secondary to rheumatic fever.

Imaging Signs

▶ **Modality of choice**
Echocardiography.

▶ **Chest radiograph findings**
Aortic configuration of the cardiac silhouette with a rounded apex (myocardial hypertrophy is demonstrated better by CT) ● LV dilatation in decompensated cases ● Aortic ectasia or aneurysm ● Possible calcification of the aortic valve.

▶ **Echocardiographic findings**
Calcification and/or fibrosis of the aortic valve with decreased opening of the valve leaflets ● The pressure gradient and VOA can be semiquantitatively assessed by using the modified Bernoulli equation (pressure gradient [mmHg] = 4 v^2) and continuity equation ● Initially normal-sized LV with good systolic function ● Myocardial hypertrophy.

▶ **MRI findings**
Not indicated in most cases ● Findings same as echocardiography, but MRI more clearly defines the adjacent vessels ● Hemodynamic significance can be determined by flow quantification (phase-velocity mapping) or VOA planimetry ● Accurate assessment of myocardial hypertrophy.

Fig. 3.1 High-grade aortic stenosis (VOA 0.8 cm²). Preoperative P-A chest radiograph shows the aortic configuration of the cardiac silhouette with a rounded apex and LV enlargement (arrows). The ascending aorta shows ectatic elongation and forms the right border of the cardiac silhouette.

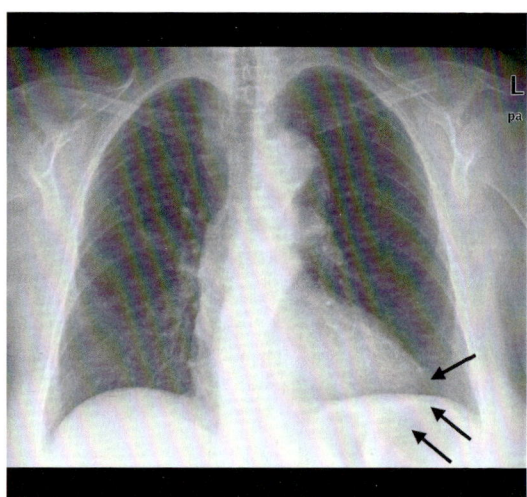

Fig. 3.2 Multidetector CT in the same patient as in Fig. 3.1 shows a calcified aortic valve and LV hypertrophy due to chronic pressure overload.

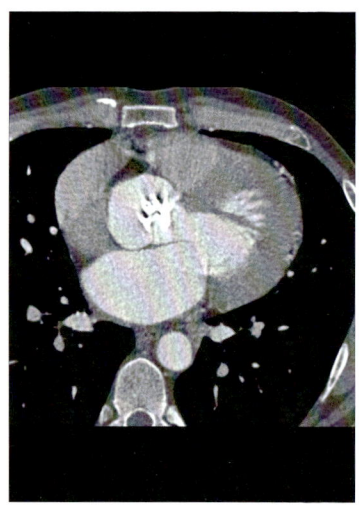

▶ **Invasive diagnostic procedures**
Coronary angiography to exclude CHD prior to valve replacement • Invasive measurement of the pressure gradient across the valve possible • Calculation of the VOA.

Clinical Aspects

▶ **Typical presentation**
Remains clinically silent for years • Many cases are diagnosed incidentally by the auscultation of a systolic murmur • Symptomatic aortic stenosis has three clinical hallmarks: angina pectoris, syncope, and dyspnea.

▶ **Treatment options**
Treatment of choice is aortic valve replacement • It is indicated for severe aortic stenosis (VOA < 1 cm²) • An alternative in young patients with congenital aortic stenosis is balloon valvuloplasty.

▶ **Course and prognosis**
Good in asymptomatic patients • Life expectancy of symptomatic patients without valve replacement is 2–5 years, depending on clinical severity (see above) • Early mortality rate is 2–8%.

▶ **What does the clinician want to know?**
Degree of severity of aortic stenosis • VOA • Myocardial hypertrophy and LV function • Aortic pathology.

Differential Diagnosis

Other valvular disease	– Aortic insufficiency
	– Mitral stenosis
	– Combined valvular disease
Myocardial hypertrophy	– Arterial hypertension
	– HCM
	– Uremic cardiomyopathy
	– Other secondary cardiomyopathies

Tips and Pitfalls

A common error is to underestimate the hemodynamic significance of aortic stenosis on the basis of the morphologic imaging features alone.

Selected References

Palta S et al. New insights into the progression of aortic stenosis: implications for secondary prevention. Circulation 2000; 101: 2497–2502

Rahimtoola SH. Severe aortic stenosis with low systolic gradient: the good and bad news. Circulation 2000; 101: 1892–1894

Definition

▶ **Epidemiology**

Second most common valvular disease after mitral stenosis • May be acute or chronic.

Grading of severity is based on the regurgitant fraction:
- Grade I   < 15 %
- Grade II   15–30 %
- Grade III 31–50 %
- Grade IV   > 50 %

▶ **Etiology, pathophysiology, pathogenesis**

Incomplete valve closure leads to regurgitation into the LV in diastole • This leads to volume overload, dilatation, and increased stroke volume • Caused by disease of the valve leaflets (primary aortic insufficiency) or aortic root (secondary aortic insufficiency).

Acute aortic insufficiency: Infectious endocarditis (more common than in other valvular diseases) • Aortic dissection • Thoracic trauma.

Chronic aortic insufficiency: Degenerative vascular and connective tissue diseases (approximately 60 %) • Congenital heart diseases (e.g., bicuspid aortic valve, approximately 28 %) • Inflammatory diseases (endocarditis, collagen diseases, etc., approximately 15 %).

Imaging Signs

▶ **Modality of choice**

Echocardiography.

▶ **Echocardiographic findings**

Morphologic changes in the valve cusps (thickening, sclerosis, vegetations) • Regurgitation jet on color Doppler scan • Semiquantitative grading of aortic insufficiency severity • LV dilatation with a normal EF • Possible myocardial hypertrophy or aortic ectasia • Late stage marked by severe structural dilatation and LV dysfunction • Secondary mitral insufficiency.

▶ **Chest radiograph and CT findings**

LV dilatation • Ectasia of the ascending aorta • LA dilatation and chronic congestive signs may be seen in decompensated aortic insufficiency • Precise visualization of the thoracic aorta • Valve morphology can be evaluated by ECG-gated multidetector CT.

▶ **MRI findings**

Same as CT findings • Also yields functional information • Regurgitant jet appears as infravalvular diastolic signal void in the blood current (turbulent flow) • Quantification of LV function (EDV, EF) and regurgitant fraction (flow measurement by phase-contrast imaging).

▶ **Invasive diagnostic procedures**

Left heart catheterization preoperatively to exclude CHD • Determination of the pressure gradient across the aortic valve (to exclude combined valvular disease).

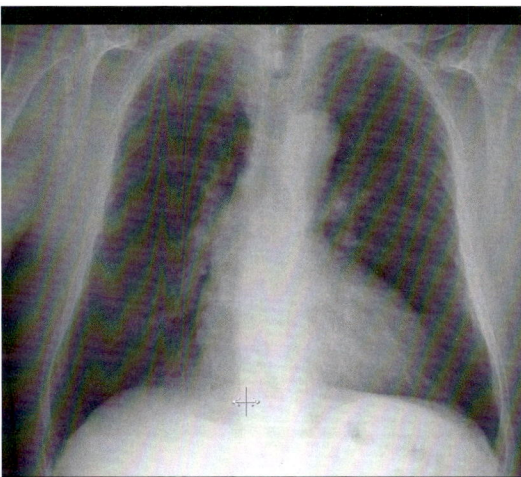

Fig. 3.3 Grade III aortic insufficiency. P-A chest radiograph shows a typical configuration of the cardiac silhouette with LV dilatation in response to chronic volume overload. The ascending aorta is ectatic and forms the right border of the cardiac silhouette.

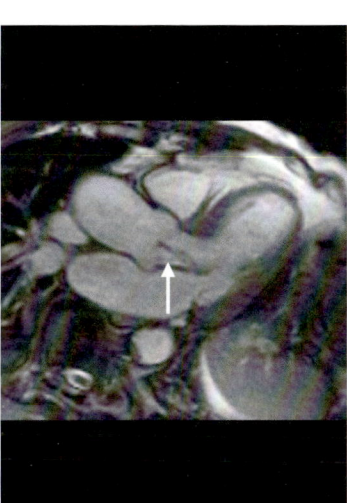

Fig. 3.4 MR image of the same patient as in Fig. 3.**3**. SSFP sequence of the LVOT (three-chamber view) shows a central regurgitant jet (arrow) across the aortic valve. The jet extends to the anterior mitral valve leaflet (may be audible as an Austin–Flint murmur).

Clinical Aspects

▶ **Typical presentation**

Remains clinically silent for years • Typical water-hammer pulse (high pulse rate with high pressure amplitudes) • Subsequent exertional dyspnea • Paroxysmal nocturnal dyspnea and orthopnea • Angina pectoris is less common than in aortic stenosis • Acute aortic insufficiency is marked by reflex tachycardia and pulmonary congestion.

▶ **Treatment options**

Initial pharmacologic treatment as for heart failure • β-blockers should be avoided as they prolong diastole and are negatively inotropic! • Eventual surgical valve replacement.

▶ **Course and prognosis**

Very good in asymptomatic patients • Up to 2% of patients per year develop LV dysfunction • Annual mortality rate among patients with angina pectoris is up to 10% • Reaches 20% in patients with symptoms of heart failure • Prognosis improves with early operative treatment.

▶ **What does the clinician want to know?**

Hemodynamic significance of the aortic insufficiency (regurgitant fraction, LV dilatation, EF) • Aortic disease • Myocardial hypertrophy • Secondary mitral insufficiency • Signs of heart failure such as pulmonary congestion or edema.

Differential Diagnosis

Diseases of the aortic root	– Aortic ectasia
	– Aortic aneurysm
	– Aortic dissection
	– Marfan syndrome
Bicuspid aortic valve	– Incomplete valve closure
	– Predisposition to endocarditis
Rheumatoid diseases	– Inflammatory and degenerative changes in the valve apparatus

Tips and Pitfalls

MRI may show obvious flow phenomena even in hemodynamically nonsignificant valvular disease. Thus, the significance of aortic insufficiency should be evaluated based on objective parameters such as LV function and the regurgitant fraction.

Selected References

Givehchian M et al. Aortic root remodeling: functional MRI as an accurate tool for complete follow-up. Thorac Cardiov Surg 2005; 53: 267–273

Dujardin KS etal. Mortality and morbidity of aortic regurgitation in clinical practice. A long-term follow-up study. Circulation 1999 13; 99: 1851–1857

Definition

▶ **Epidemiology**
Almost all cases (99%) are secondary to rheumatic fever • Two-thirds of patients are female • 50% of patients have combined valvular disease.

▶ **Etiology, pathophysiology, pathogenesis**
Rheumatic fever leads to fusion of the valve leaflets or commissures. Fibrosis and calcifications may spread to the valve ring and chordae tendineae. As the VOA dwindles (normal = $4-5$ cm^2), a pressure gradient develops between the LA and LV, causing decreased diastolic filling of the LV • Elevated LA pressure • Increased pressure in the pulmonary circuit ranging from pulmonary hypertension to right ventricular decompensation.
Grading of severity is based on the VOA:
- 1.5–2.5 cm^2 Mild mitral stenosis
- 1.0–1.5 cm^2 Moderate mitral stenosis
- 0.75–1 cm^2 Severe mitral stenosis
- < 0.75 cm^2 Critical mitral stenosis

Imaging Signs

▶ **Modality of choice**
Echocardiography.

▶ **Echocardiographic findings**
Thickening of the mitral valve leaflets • Planimetric or Doppler determination of severity (maximum and mean pressure gradients) • Dilatation of the LA • Evaluation of all cardiac chambers • Signs of right heart overload (or enlargement) • Functional impairment • May detect a thrombus in the LA.

▶ **Chest radiograph and CT findings**
Enlargement of the LA (central shadow, splaying of the tracheal bifurcation) • Prominent pulmonary segment • Chronic pulmonary congestion (Kerley lines) • Possible valve calcification • Cardiomegaly and pleural effusion in patients with overt right heart decompensation.

▶ **MRI findings**
Usually not indicated • Same findings as echocardiography.

▶ **Invasive diagnostic procedures**
Invasive pressure measurement can resolve discrepancy between clinical and Echocardiographic findings • Some cases require investigation by right and left heart catheterization during exercise • Preoperative coronary angiography in patients over age 45 to exclude CHD • Interventional therapy may be required (balloon valvuloplasty).

Fig. 3.5 Mitral stenosis in a 64-year-old woman. P-A chest radiograph shows a mitral configuration of the cardiac silhouette with marked dilatation of the LA (carinal angle!) and obliteration of the cardiac waist. Other findings are chronic pulmonary congestion (Kerley B lines) and pronounced right ventricular dilatation.

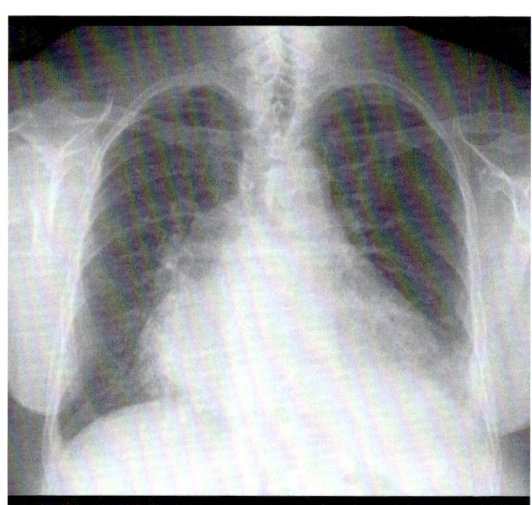

Fig. 3.6 Transthoracic echocardiography shows marked thickening of the mitral valve leaflets in the parasternal short-axis view with severe reduction in VOA (from Böhmeke T, Doliva R. *Pocket Atlas of Echocardiography.* Stuttgart: Thieme; 2006).

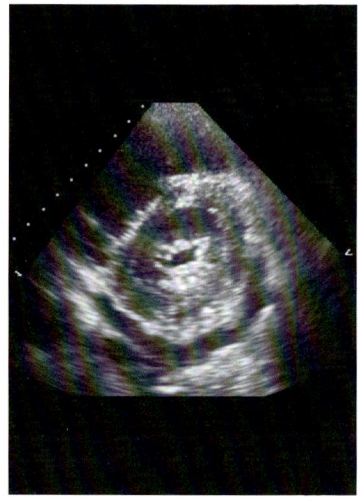

Clinical Aspects

▶ **Typical presentation**

Decreased exercise tolerance • Exertional dyspnea • Orthopnea • Hemoptysis due to acute pulmonary congestion • Mitral facies (plum-colored flush on cheeks) • Angina pectoris in 25 % of cases.

▶ **Treatment options**

Atrial fibrillation is treated medically or by electrical cardioversion • Medical stabilization of heart failure, if present • Anticoagulation for LA thrombi • Endocarditis prophylaxis may be required • Percutaneous balloon valvuloplasty (method of choice in selected patients) • Mitral valve reconstruction • Mechanical or bioprosthetic mitral valve replacement.

▶ **Course and prognosis**

Initial cardiac symptoms often postdate rheumatic fever by two to three decades • Progressive heart failure occurs in two-thirds of patients • 50 % of patients have atrial fibrillation with thromboembolic complications.

▶ **What does the clinician want to know?**

Degree of stenosis • Atrial dilatation • Thrombi • Sequelae (pulmonary hypertension, pulmonary edema) • Cardiac function • Right heart overload.

Differential Diagnosis

Infectious endocarditis	– Valvular vegetations hamper valve opening
Left atrial myxoma	– Mechanical obstruction to ventricular filling
Triatrial heart	– Accessory atrial chamber

Tips and Pitfalls

The degree of severity, optimum therapeutic approach, and optimum timing of treatment should be carefully (not always easy) determined • *Caution:* Left atrial thrombi may be a source of recurrent emboli.

Selected References

Nishimura RA et al. Accurate measurement of the transmitral gradient in patients with mitral stenosis: a simultaneous catheterization and Doppler echocardiographic study. J Am Coll Cardiol 1994; 24: 152–158

Rahimtoola SH et al. Current evaluation and management of patients with mitral stenosis. Circulation 2002; 106: 1183–1188

Definition

▶ **Epidemiology**
Usually acquired, rarely congenital • 50% of cases are based on mitral valve prolapse.

▶ **Pathoanatomy, classification**
Mitral insufficiency may be acute or chronic.
Grading of severity is based on the regurgitant fraction:
– Grade I   < 15%
– Grade II   15–30%
– Grade III   30–50%
– Grade IV   > 50%
Another option is echocardiographic grading, based on the "area" of the regurgitant jet as determined by color Doppler.

▶ **Etiology, pathophysiology, pathogenesis**
Acute mitral insufficiency: Bacterial endocarditis • Inflammatory or traumatic destruction • Degenerative • Ischemic (papillary muscle rupture due to myocardial infarction).
Chronic mitral insufficiency: Mitral valve prolapse • Papillary muscle dysfunction due to CHD • Rheumatic or infectious endocarditis • Secondary to LV dilatation (including dilated cardiomyopathies, CHD, myocarditis, and aortic anomalies).

Imaging Signs

▶ **Modality of choice**
Echocardiography.

▶ **Echocardiographic findings**
LA and LV enlargement • Morphology of the valve leaflets • Vegetations • Grading of severity by color Doppler.

▶ **Chest radiograph and CT findings**
Dilatation of the LA and LV • Obliterated cardiac waist with a mitral configuration of the cardiac silhouette • Possible signs of chronic congestion • Indentation or displacement of the esophagus • Mitral valve calcification • Valve morphology can be evaluated by ECG-gated multidetector CT.

▶ **MRI findings**
Same findings as CT • Also supplies functional information • Systolic regurgitant jet directed toward the LA (turbulent flow) • LV function (EDV, EF) and regurgitant fraction can be quantified by comparing the RV and LV stroke volumes.

▶ **Invasive diagnostic procedures**
Primary left heart catheterization to exclude CHD before surgery • Left ventriculogram to demonstrate the mitral insufficiency • Right heart catheterization to determine the PA and PC pressure • Exclusion of combined valvular disease.

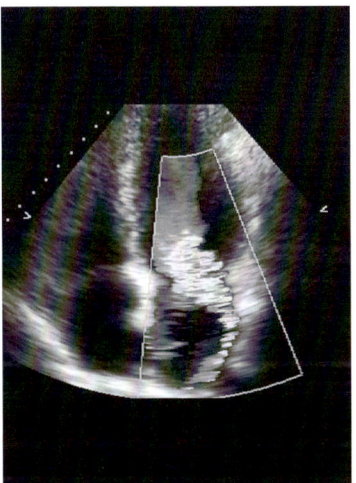

Fig. 3.7 Mitral insufficiency. Echocardiogram shows significant regurgitation into the left atrium through the centrally incompetent mitral valve (from Böhmeke T, Doliva R. *Pocket Atlas of Echocardiography.* Stuttgart: Thieme; 2006).

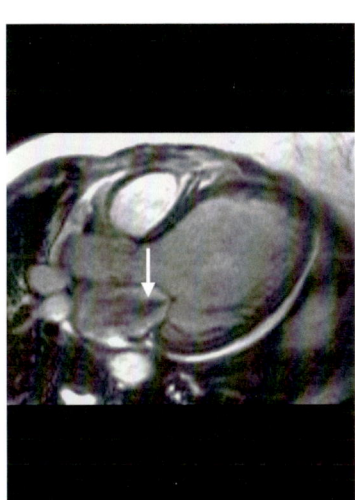

Fig. 3.8 MR image of mitral insufficiency. SSFP sequence in the four-chamber view shows a central systolic regurgitant jet across the mitral valve (arrow) with pronounced LV dilatation.

Clinical Aspects

▶ **Typical presentation**
Acute mitral insufficiency: Signs of acute heart failure ranging from pulmonary edema to cardiogenic shock.
Chronic mitral insufficiency: Prolonged absence of complaints • Possible atrial fibrillation • Signs and symptoms of heart failure in decompensated cases.

▶ **Treatment options**
Secondary mitral insufficiency requires pharmacologic treatment for heart failure and the underlying disease • Surgical reconstruction or replacement of the mitral valve.

▶ **Course and prognosis**
Even severe mitral insufficiency may remain asymptomatic for years • Symptom onset is marked by decreased LV function, LV dilatation, and/or pulmonary hypertension; patients then should be evaluated for surgery.

▶ **What does the clinician want to know?**
Dilatation of the LA and LV • Ventricular function (EF) • Degree of insufficiency (echo) • Signs of heart failure.

Differential Diagnosis

Infectious endocarditis	– Acute mitral insufficiency due to valve destruction
Other heart diseases	– DCM and advanced CHD: LV dilatation with secondary dilatation of the mitral ring

Tips and Pitfalls

It can be difficult to determine the hemodynamic significance of mitral insufficiency and the optimum timing of operative treatment • Several modalities (echocardiography and MRI or invasive imaging) may be necessary in addition to the clinical assessment.

Selected References

Kon MW et al. Quantification of regurgitant fraction in mitral regurgitation by cardiovascular magnetic resonance: comparison of techniques. J Heart Valve Dis 2004; 13: 600–607

Kouris N et al. Mitral valve repair versus replacement for isolated non-ischemic mitral regurgitation in patients with preoperative left ventricular dysfunction. A long-term follow-up echocardiography study. Eur J Echocardiogr 2005; 6: 435–442

Definition

▶ **Epidemiology**
Almost always congenital (9% of all cardiac anomalies) • Usually combined with other anomalies (21% of all heart defects, e.g., ASD, VSD, tetralogy of Fallot) • Very rarely acquired.

▶ **Etiology, pathophysiology, pathogenesis**
Congenital fusion of the valve cusps or postinflammatory or neoplastic processes (carcinoid) lead to a reduction of VOA • This leads to rise in RV pressure • Isolated pulmonary stenosis leads to RV hypertrophy (pressure overload).

▶ **Classification**
Grading of severity is based on the pressure gradient:
– 25–49 mmHg   Mild pulmonary stenosis
– 50–79 mmHg   Moderate pulmonary stenosis
– > 80 mmHg   Severe to critical pulmonary stenosis

Imaging Signs

▶ **Modality of choice**
Echocardiography.

▶ **Chest radiograph and CT findings**
Initially normal • Subsequent signs of RV and pulmonary artery dilatation • Possible signs of right-sided heart failure (inflow stasis, pleural effusion) • CT accurately defines the pulmonary arterial tract.

▶ **Echocardiography findings**
Restriction of pulmonary valve opening • Systolic doming of the pulmonary valve • Degree of severity can be quantified with color Doppler by estimating the pressure gradient based on maximum flow velocity (modified Bernoulli equation) • Poststenotic dilatation of the pulmonary artery.

▶ **MRI findings**
Same as echocardiography findings • Used mainly to investigate congenital anomalies • Systolic flow void across the pulmonary valve • Can exclude extrinsic compression or mechanical obstruction (subvalvular hypertrophy).

▶ **Invasive diagnostic procedures**
Within the context of treatment, e.g., for invasive pressure measurements • Indicated mainly for congenital valve disease.

Clinical Aspects

▶ **Typical presentation**
Remains asymptomatic for years • Late stages are marked by angina pectoris and exertional dyspnea.

Fig. 3.9 Pulmonary stenosis. Echocardiogram shows valvular pulmonary stenosis with typical doming in a modified short-axis view (from Flachskampf FA. *Kursbuch Echokardiographie*. Stuttgart: Thieme; 2004).

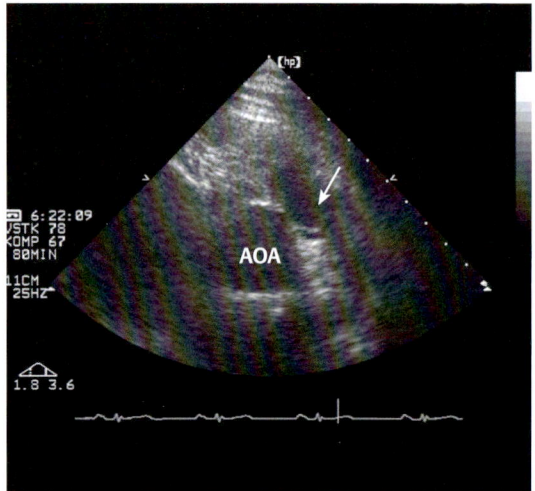

Fig. 3.10 Magnified view. The valve leaflets are relatively thin (from Flachskampf FA. *Kursbuch Echokardiographie*. Stuttgart: Thieme; 2004).

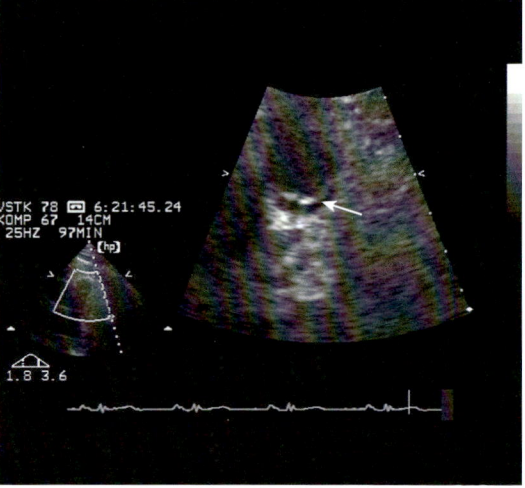

▶ **Treatment options**
Medical treatment for right-sided heart failure if the pressure gradient is less than 50 mmHg • Percutaneous balloon valvuloplasty is the procedure of choice in adolescents and young adults • Operative correction is usually combined with other surgical measures.

▶ **Course and prognosis**
Life expectancy is not significantly reduced in the absence of pulmonary hypertension • Increased risk of paradoxical emboli through a patent foramen ovale.

▶ **What does the clinician want to know?**
Quantification of the pulmonary stenosis • Right heart function • Myocardial hypertrophy • RV dilatation • Status of pulmonary vessels • Signs of right-sided heart failure.

Differential Diagnosis

Rheumatic fever	– Frequent degenerative calcification of multiple valves (mitral stenosis, aortic stenosis)
Congenital heart defects	– Associated with other complex anomalies such as ASD, VSD, and tetralogy of Fallot

Tips and Pitfalls

Pulmonary stenosis in carcinoid syndrome often occurs in combination with tricuspid valve disease.

Selected References

Earing MG. Long-term follow-up of patients after surgical treatment for isolated pulmonary valve stenosis. Mayo Clin Proc 2005; 80: 871–876

Silvilairat S. Echocardiographic assessment of isolated pulmonary valve stenosis: which outpatient Doppler gradient has the most clinical validity? J Am Soc Echocardiogr 2005; 18: 1137–1142

Definition

▶ **Epidemiology**
A rare disease.
▶ **Etiology, pathophysiology, pathogenesis**
Dilatation of the pulmonary valve ring • RV volume overload.

Imaging Signs

▶ **Modality of choice**
Echocardiography.
▶ **Chest radiograph and CT findings**
Dilatation of the right heart (RV + RA) • Dilatation of the pulmonary artery (prominent pulmonary segment with opacification of much of the retrosternal space in the lateral radiograph) • Left ventricle is displaced laterally and posteriorly • Possible signs of primary lung disease as cause of pulmonary hypertension • CT accurately defines the pulmonary arterial tract.
▶ **Echocardiography findings**
Degree of insufficiency can be quantified with color Doppler • Dilatation of the RV and RA • Myocardial hypertrophy in pulmonary hypertension • Possible decrease in EF and secondary tricuspid insufficiency • Rapid diastolic fluttering movement of the anterior tricuspid valve leaflet • Possible valvular vegetations.
▶ **MRI findings**
Findings same as echocardiography and CT findings • Used mainly in patients with secondary pulmonary insufficiency in the workup of congenital anomalies • Quantification of flow (phase-velocity mapping) to determine the regurgitant fraction.
▶ **Invasive diagnostic procedures**
Necessary only in cases requiring more detailed investigation (invasive pressure measurements; association with congenital anomalies, see below).

Clinical Aspects

▶ **Typical presentation**
Patients with acquired pulmonary valve disease are largely free of complaints • Only patients with progressive pulmonary insufficiency show signs of right-sided heart failure.
▶ **Treatment options**
Initial medical treatment for pulmonary hypertension and right-sided heart failure • Rare cases (e.g., following the correction of Fallot tetralogy) will require valve replacement with a bioprosthesis or allograft.
▶ **Course and prognosis**
The prognosis depends on the underlying disease and condition of the right heart.

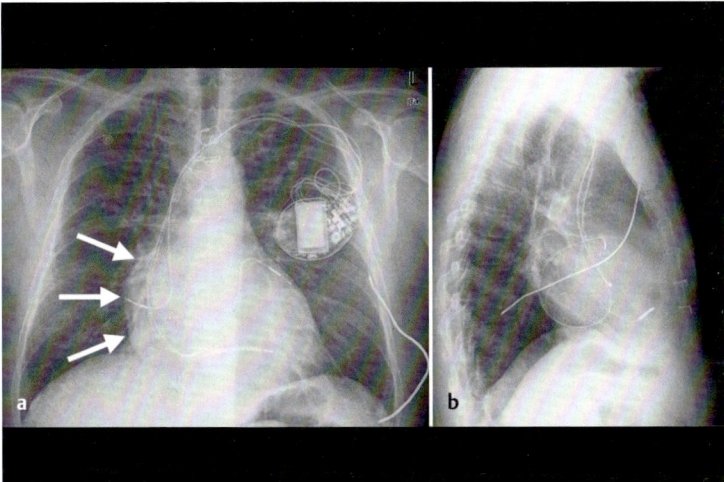

Fig. 3.11   Pulmonary insufficiency. P-A and lateral chest radiographs show dilatation of the right ventricle and atrium with associated widening of the cardiac silhouette (arrows). Note the implanted cardiac defibrillator.

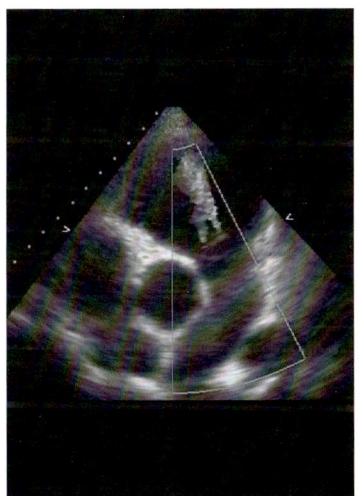

Fig. 3.12   Duplex echocardiogram in pulmonary insufficiency shows a regurgitant jet over the pulmonary valve extending to the center of the RV (from Böhmeke T, Doliva R. *Pocket Atlas of Echocardiography.* Stuttgart: Thieme; 2006).

▶ **What does the clinician want to know?**
Severity of pulmonary insufficiency ● Signs of chronic volume overload (RV hypertrophy, RV dilatation) ● Right-sided heart failure (inflow stasis, hepatomegaly).

Differential Diagnosis

Congenital valvular disease	– Congenital malformations or pulmonary valve insufficiency
	– Often combined with other cardiac anomalies

Tips and Pitfalls

Always investigate and treat the underlying disease in patients with pulmonary insufficiency.

Selected References

Doughan AR et al. Effects of pulmonary valve replacement on QRS duration and right ventricular cavity size late after repair of right ventricular outflow tract obstruction. Am J Cardiol 2005; 95: 1511–1514

Therrien J et al. Optimal timing for pulmonary valve replacement in adults after tetralogy of Fallot repair. Am J Cardiol 2005; 95: 779–782

Definition

▶ **Epidemiology**
Usually develops in a setting of rheumatic fever ● Less common than an isolated acquired defect (up to 7% of all patients with rheumatic fever; more common in females than in males [3:2]) ● Commonly associated with mitral and aortic valve disease.

▶ **Pathogenesis, pathophysiology**
Inflammatory contracture of the chordae tendinae ● Shrinkage and fusion of the valve leaflets and commissures ● Valve calcifications are unusual ● Tricuspid stenosis is present when the VOA is less than 2 cm^2 (normal = $6-8 \text{ cm}^2$) ● Severe tricuspid stenosis is present when the pressure gradient reaches 7 mmHg.

Imaging Signs

▶ **Modality of choice**
Echocardiography.

▶ **Chest radiograph and CT findings**
Widening of the RA ● Cardiomegaly may result from involvement of additional heart valves ● Dilatation of the superior vena cava and azygos vein ● Valvular calcification is rare.

▶ **Echocardiography findings**
Restricted valve opening with thickening of the valve leaflets (best demonstrated by TEE) ● *Pathognomonic sign:* diastolic doming and decreased excursions of the valve leaflets ● Dilatation of the RA, venae cavae, and hepatic veins ● Color Doppler can grade the degree of stenosis and estimate the pressure gradient.

▶ **MRI findings**
Not indicated in tricuspid stenosis ● Tricuspid stenosis is occasionally detected incidentally on MRI ● These changes resemble echocardiography findings ● Stenotic jet appears as a systolic artifact of low signal intensity.

▶ **Invasive diagnostic procedures**
No immediate indications ● Coronary angiography is done to exclude CHD before operative treatment.

Clinical Aspects

▶ **Typical presentation**
Cases with normal pressure relationships remain asymptomatic for many years ● Eventual signs of superior and inferior vena caval obstruction ● Dyspnea ● Decreased exercise tolerance ● Peripheral cyanosis.

▶ **Treatment options**
Medical treatment of right-sided heart failure ● Good results are achieved with balloon valvuloplasty ● Alternative is valve reconstruction or replacement (preferably with a bioprosthesis).

Fig. 3.13 Acquired tricuspid stenosis in a 38-year-old man with a history of rheumatic fever. P-A chest radiograph showing enlarged RA. The patient presented clinically with dyspnea on exertion and distended neck veins.

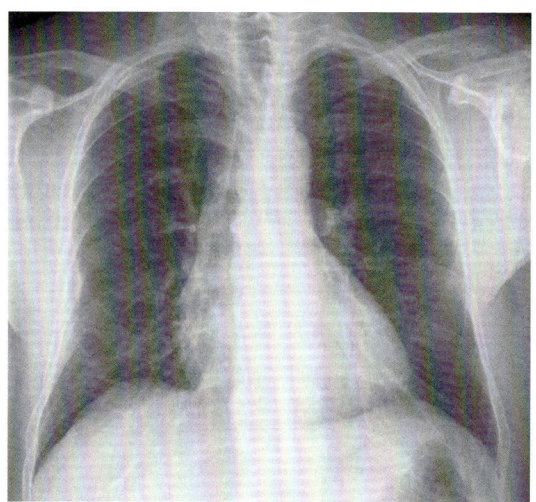

Fig. 3.14 Tricuspid stenosis. Echocardiogram (four-chamber view) shows thickening and doming of the tricuspid valve leaflets (arrow) with an enlarged RA (from Flachskampf FA. *Kursbuch Echokardiographie*. Stuttgart: Thieme; 2004).

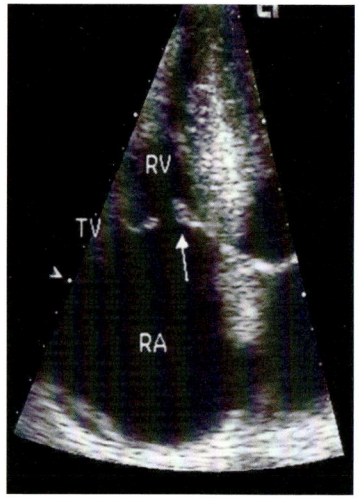

▶ **Course and prognosis**

Secondary organ changes (liver and renal failure) are the dominant features in patients with isolated tricuspid stenosis • Associated aortic and mitral valve disease usually determine the prognosis • Long-term survival rates after tricuspid valve replacement: 70% at 5 years, 55% at 10 years.

▶ **What does the clinician want to know?**

Degree of severity of the tricuspid stenosis • Associated valvular disease • Atrial dilatation • Thrombi • RV function • Sequelae (inflow stasis, hepatomegaly, ascites).

Differential Diagnosis

Right atrial masses	– Myxoma, metastasis
	– Thrombi that narrow the tricuspid orifice

Tips and Pitfalls

Because isolated tricuspid stenosis is very rare, all heart valves should be closely scrutinized in patients with a history of rheumatic fever.

Selected References

Chockalingam A et al. Clinical spectrum of chronic rheumatic heart disease in India. J Heart Valve Dis 2003; 12: 577–581

Goswami KC et al. Juvenile tricuspid stenosis and rheumatic tricuspid valve disease: an echocardiographic study. Int J Cardiol 1999; 72: 83–86

Definition

▶ **Epidemiology**
Very rare as an isolated condition.

▶ **Etiology, pathophysiology, pathogenesis**
Tricuspid insufficiency can be a consequence of dilatation of the valvular ring •
Primary tricuspid insufficiency results from a malformed valve (e.g., Ebstein
anomaly, tricuspid valve prolapse in 20% of patients with mitral valve prolapse,
Marfan syndrome) • Acquired tricuspid insufficiency may be secondary to rheu-
matic fever, endocarditis, cor pulmonale, or left ventricular decompensation •
Secondary tricuspid insufficiency is more common.

Imaging Signs

▶ **Modality of choice**
Echocardiography.

▶ **Chest radiograph and CT findings**
Enlargement of the RA and RV • Increased pulmonary vascular markings are
seen in patients with LV decompensation • Chronic congestion and cardiomegaly may occur • Prominent venae cavae and azygos vein.

▶ **Echocardiography findings**
Evaluation of valve morphology • Dilatation of the RA and RV • Tricuspid insufficiency can be visualized and graded with color Doppler • Severe tricuspid insufficiency is present when the area of the regurgitant jet exceeds 8 cm^2 • Severe
tricuspid insufficiency is associated with dilatation and reversal of flow in the
hepatic veins and loss of respiratory flow modulation in the inferior vena cava •
Echocardiography can assess pulmonary arterial pressure in suspected cases of
secondary tricuspid insufficiency (pressure gradient > 55 mmHg).

▶ **MRI findings**
Generally not indicated • Tricuspid insufficiency may be an associated or incidental finding in other cardiac diseases.

▶ **Invasive diagnostic procedures**
Generally not indicated • Can be done to determine right cardiac and pulmonary
arterial pressures.

Clinical Aspects

▶ **Typical presentation**
Initially nonspecific symptoms (decreased exercise tolerance, arrhythmias) •
With the development of right-sided heart failure, congestive signs appear (he-
patic congestion, portal hypertension, ascites).

▶ **Treatment options**
Secondary tricuspid insufficiency warrants causal treatment of the underlying
disease • Medical stabilization of right-sided heart failure • Isolated tricuspid
valve reconstruction or replacement (preferably with an annuloplasty ring or
bioprosthesis), depending on valve condition and etiology.

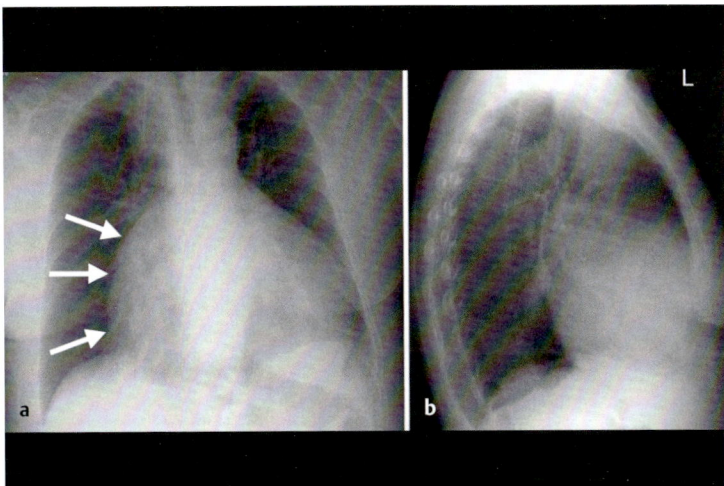

Fig. 3.15 a, b Secondary tricuspid insufficiency in left-sided heart failure. P-A (**a**) and lateral chest radiograph (**b**) show cardiomegaly with marked enlargement of the LA and LV and opacification of the retrosternal space by the RV. Pulmonary venous congestion is moderate in relation to cardiac size. A CVC is also present.

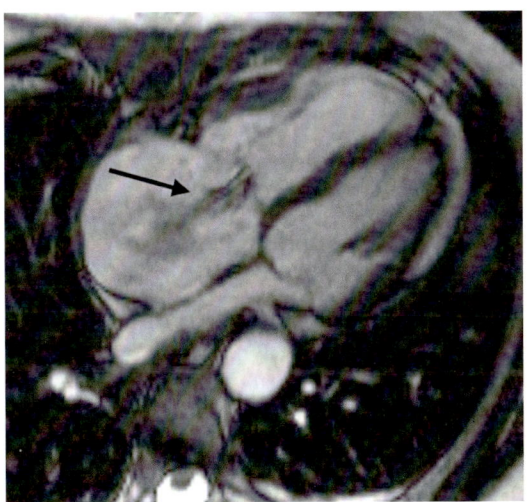

Fig. 3.16 Tricuspid insufficiency (incidental MRI finding) in a 60-year-old man. SSFP sequence in the four-chamber view shows a regurgitant jet across the tricuspid valve during systole (arrow).

▶ **Course and prognosis**

Remains asymptomatic for years in the absence of pulmonary hypertension •
Prognosis of secondary tricuspid insufficiency is determined by the underlying
disease.

▶ **What does the clinician want to know?**

Morphology of the cardiac chambers • Degree of severity of tricuspid insufficiency • Signs of right-sided heart failure (vena cava, hepatic veins, ascites, edema).

Differential Diagnosis

Ebstein anomaly	– Congenital anomaly marked by displacement of a malformed tricuspid valve into the right ventricle, leading to "atrialization" of the upper portion of the RV; secondary tricuspid insufficiency
Infectious endocarditis	– Degeneration and fibrosis of the valve cusps.
Iatrogenic injury	– Injury to the valve apparatus from a pacemaker lead or right-heart catheter.

Tips and Pitfalls

Many common disorders can lead to secondary tricuspid insufficiency. This should
always be considered in diagnosing the underlying disease.

Selected References

Frater R. Tricuspid insufficiency. J Thorac Cardiovasc Surg 2001; 122: 427–429

Mueller XM et al. Tricuspid valve involvement in combined mitral and aortic valve surgery. J Cardiovasc Surg 2001; 42: 443–449

Definition

▶ **Epidemiology**
Chronic forms of acquired valvular disease often lead to combined aortic and mitral valve defects • Combined valvular diseases occur predominantly in older patients • Up to 30% of mitral valve defects are combined forms (50% isolated stenosis, 20% isolated insufficiency) • Males are predisposed to combined aortic valve disease • Females are more prone to combined mitral valve disease.

▶ **Etiology, pathophysiology, pathogenesis**
Usually has a degenerative cause • Rheumatic and infectious causes are less common • The combination of stenosis and insufficiency can lead to left heart decompensation • One of the two lesions is hemodynamically predominant in most cases (e.g., aortic stenosis in patients with combined aortic stenosis and aortic insufficiency).

Imaging Signs

▶ **Modality of choice**
Echocardiography.

▶ **Chest radiograph and CT findings**
Findings depend on the dominant valve lesion • Left heart decompensation is not uncommon • This is followed by LV dilatation and acute or chronic congestion (pulmonary edema, Kerley lines, pleural effusion) • Decompensated aortic valve disease is marked by aortic ectasia or aneurysm • Calcification of one or more heart valves.

▶ **Echocardiography findings**
Thickening and impaired function of the aortic or mitral valve, depending on the underlying disease • LV dilatation • Myocardial hypertrophy • Decreased EF • Color Doppler is of limited value for assessing the stenotic gradient or regurgitant fraction.

▶ **MRI findings**
Same as echocardiography findings • Stenotic or regurgitant jet can be identified as a hypointense flow artifact in cine sequences • Quantification of flow (phase-velocity mapping) or comparison of right and left stroke volumes to determine hemodynamic significance

Clinical Aspects

▶ **Typical presentation**
The clinical presentation is usually determined by the dominant lesion • This often delays the diagnosis of combined valvular disease • Combined lesions can lead to left ventricular decompensation, even if the dominant lesion is not severe.

Fig. 3.17 A 58-year-old man with a long history of known aortic stenosis. MR image, SSFP sequence (three-chamber view), shows marked thickening of the aortic valve and a supravalvular stenotic jet during systole (arrow).

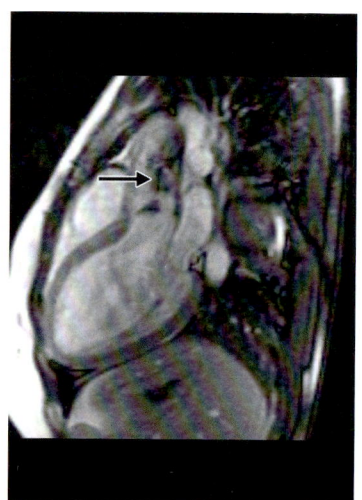

Fig. 3.18 Same patient as in Fig. 3.**17**. SSFP sequence in the plane of the LVOT (three-chamber view) shows a diastolic regurgitant jet (arrow) extending to the mitral valve leaflet.

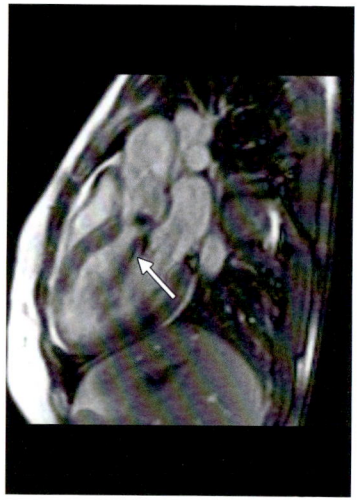

▶ **Treatment options**

Individual treatment planning is required ● The only surgical option is valve re-placement ● Surgical mortality is markedly higher than with isolated valve dis-ease (5–10%, depending on patient's age).

▶ **Course and prognosis**

When clinical manifestations are present, in most patients the LV myocardium will already be irreversibly damaged ● Combined mitral valve disease often leads to early atrial fibrillation with risk of thromboembolism ● Systemic antico-agulation is required.

▶ **What does the clinician want to know?**

Dilatation of the right or left heart ● Myocardial hypertrophy ● Secondary valvu-lar disease ● Valvular morphology.

Differential Diagnosis
....

Isolated valvular disease   – Aortic valve: systolic stenotic jet or diastolic regurgitant jet

Tips and Pitfalls
....

Echocardiography and invasive diagnostic procedures are of limited value for quan-tifying the stenotic or regurgitant component in patients with combined valvular disease. Therefore flow quantification by MRI is a valuable alternative. It should be used whenever a discrepancy is noted between clinical and imaging findings.

Selected References

Lethen H, Lambertz H. Transösophageale Echokardiographie. Stuttgart: Thieme; 2000

Lotz J et al. Cardiovascular flow measurement with phase-contrast MR imaging: basic facts and implementation. Radiographics 2002; 22: 651–671

Definition

▶ **Definition, epidemiology**

Excessive bulging of the mitral valve leaflets into the LA during systole • Overall prevalence is approximately 2% • Approximately 4% of affected patients have hemodynamically significant MVP.

▶ **Pathoanatomy, classification**

Systolic prolapse of the mitral valve leaflets > 2 mm (echocardiography) • *Synonyms:* Barlow syndrome, floppy-valve syndrome.

▶ **Etiology, pathophysiology, pathogenesis**

Primary mitral valve prolapse: Hereditary connective tissue disease of unknown etiology • Typically associated with myxoid thickening to more than 5 mm • Also found in Marfan and Ehlers–Danlos syndromes, osteogenesis imperfecta, etc. • Other causes are HCM, rheumatic heart disease, CHD, and rupture of chordae tendineae • Hemodynamically significant mitral regurgitation may be present, depending on the degree of severity.

Imaging Signs

▶ **Modality of choice**

Echocardiography.

▶ **Echocardiography findings**

Prolapse of one or both leaflets or portions of the leaflets beyond the plane of the mitral valve ring into the atrium (> 2 mm) during systole • Valve morphology • Degree of severity of mitral insufficiency • Ventricular and atrial size • Myocardial function.

▶ **Chest radiograph and CT findings**

Often normal findings • Significant mitral insufficiency may produce a mitral cardiac configuration with dilatation of the LA • Indentation or displacement of the esophagus • Pulmonary venous congestion.

▶ **MRI findings**

Generally not indicated • Given its prevalence, it is not unusual to detect MVP as an incidental finding • Criteria same as echocardiography • *Caution:* Flow phenomena vary with the type of sequence used, so analysis of the regurgitant jet should be supplemented by indirect parameters (atrial size, pulmonary venous congestion) for assessment of hemodynamic significance • Function can also be quantified by comparing the RV and LV stroke volumes.

▶ **Invasive diagnostic procedures**

Not indicated.

Clinical Aspects

▶ **Typical presentation**

Usually detected incidentally in asymptomatic patients • Occasional palpitations (cardiac arrhythmias) • Heart failure • Endocarditis.

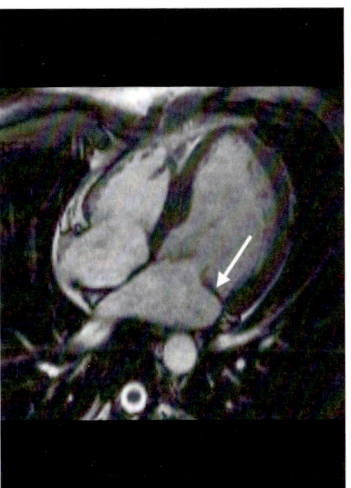

Fig. 3.19 Mitral valve prolapse. SSFP sequence in the four-chamber view during diastole shows thickening of the posterior mitral valve leaflet (arrow) with secondary MI (classified as grade II by echocardiography).

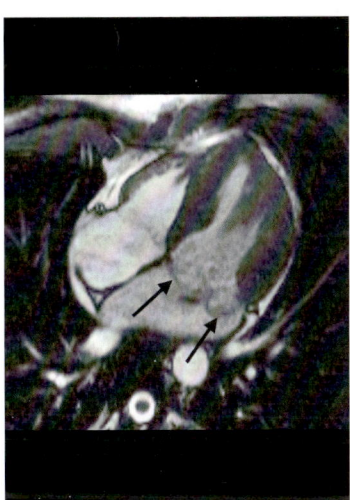

Fig. 3.20 Same patient as in Fig. 3.**19**. SSFP sequence in the four-chamber view during systole shows the mitral valve leaflets prolapsing across the plane of the mitral ring (arrows) into the left atrium.

▶ **Treatment options**

Asymptomatic patients without mitral insufficiency do not require treatment •
Patients should be followed at 3- to 5-year intervals • Symptomatic patients
should receive medical treatment for heart failure • Endocarditis prophylaxis •
Anticoagulation • Severe cases are treated by surgical valve reconstruction or replacement.

▶ **Course and prognosis**

Good • Most patients remain asymptomatic for life.

▶ **What does the clinician want to know?**

Valvular morphology and function • Degree of severity of mitral insufficiency •
Morphology of the LA and LV • Signs of heart failure.

Differential Diagnosis

Primary mitral insufficiency	– See under Mitral Insufficiency
Other causes of heart failure	– Other valvular disease
	– Secondary mitral insufficiency in CHD
	– DCM
	– Myocarditis

Tips and Pitfalls

MVP in itself does not have pathologic significance. When detected incidentally,
therefore, its hemodynamic significance should be carefully evaluated and the patient educated about the relative importance of the finding.

Selected References

David TE et al. A comparison of outcomes of mitral valve repair for degenerative disease
with posterior, anterior, and bileaflet prolapse. J Thorac Cardiovasc Surg 2005; 130:
1242–1249

Plicht B et al. Valve Prolapse: Identification of High-Risk Patients and Therapeutic Management. Herz 2006; 31: 14–21

Definition

▶ **Epidemiology**
Aortic valve replacements account for approximately 10% of all heart operations in Western countries, and double valve replacements for approximately 7% • The major indication is valvular aortic stenosis in the setting of isolated (90%) or combined (10%) valvular disease • A mechanical aortic valve prosthesis is implanted in 56% of cases.

▶ **Pathoanatomy, classification**
Prosthetic heart valves are classified into three types based on their origin:
– Mechanical valves.
– Biologic valves (e.g., excised porcine valves).
– Allografts (cadaver valves).
Mechanical valves may be implanted in isolation or may be placed in the ascending aorta as a valved conduit with reimplantation of the coronary arteries.

▶ **Etiology, pathophysiology, pathogenesis**
Biologic valves and allografts have relatively favorable hemodynamic properties • Stentless bioprostheses have the best hemodynamic properties • Mechanical valves are more thrombogenic (requiring anticoagulation) but have better durability.

Imaging Signs

▶ **Modality of choice**
Echocardiography.

▶ **Chest radiograph findings**
The configuration of the cardiac silhouette depends on the underlying valvular disease • Cardiomegaly may be present • Early postoperative cases may also show congestive signs, mediastinal widening (hematoma), pericardial or pleural effusion, and/or ventilation abnormalities • Valve prosthesis or bioprosthesis stent.

▶ **Echocardiography findings**
Evaluation of valve function • May show turbulent flow pattern • Can exclude recurrent stenosis or insufficiency with bioprostheses and allografts • Early postoperative paravalvular leak in rare cases • Slight regurgitation is normal in mechanical valves • Evaluation of ventricular function • Pericardial effusion.

▶ **CT findings**
Used mainly to investigate suspected extracardiac complications in the early postoperative period (mediastinal hematoma, lung pathology, anastomotic leak on a valved conduit) • Metallic artifacts limit the ability to evaluate valves.

▶ **MRI findings**
Caution: Older biologic valves with a metal stent may be incompatible with MRI • Newer bioprostheses use titanium alloys, which generally are MRI compatible • Always check compatibility in doubtful cases.

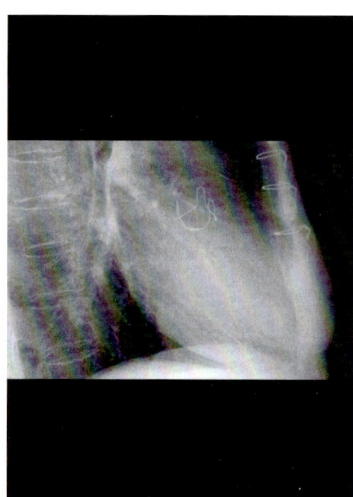

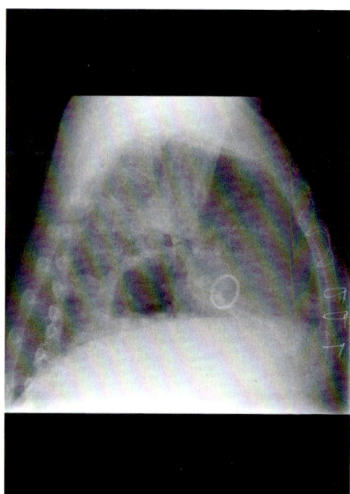

Fig. 3.21 Aortic valve replacement. Lateral chest radiograph in a 56-year-old woman who underwent a bioprosthetic aortic valve replacement. The housing of the bioprosthetic valve is visible in the aortic valve region. Sternal cerclage wires are also seen.

Fig. 3.23 Mitral valve replacement. Contrast-enhanced multidetector CT shows a metallic artifact from the mechanical prosthesis in the mitral valve region. Postoperative pleural effusion (*).

Fig. 3.22 Mitral valve replacement with a mechanical prosthesis. Lateral chest radiograph shows the valve prosthesis in the mitral valve region. Marked pericardial effusion is still present in the early postoperative period. Basal dyselectasis in the left lung with accompanying pleural effusion.

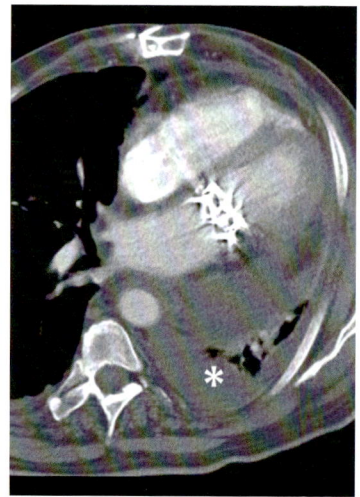

▶ **Invasive diagnostic procedures**
Patients over 45 years of age should undergo preoperative coronary angiography to exclude CHD.

Clinical Aspects

▶ **Typical presentation**
Patients are asymptomatic after postoperative convalescence • A high-frequency metallic closing sound is heard on auscultation of mechanical valves • A soft systolic murmur is occasionally audible in a functioning bioprostheses • No "valve click."

▶ **Treatment options, course and prognosis**
Biologic valves do not require anticoagulation and have better hemodynamic properties • They may degenerate under heavy mechanical loads, leading to progressive calcification with stenosis and eventual need for reoperation • Rate of reoperation at 10 years is approximately 20–30% • Mechanical valves are more durable but require lifelong anticoagulation.

Early mortality rate after aortic valve replacement is approximately 5% • Long-term survival is 75% at 5 years, 50% at 10 years, and 30% at 15 years • Patients with a valve allograft will probably require reoperation after about 15 years.

▶ **What does the clinician want to know?**
Valvular morphology • Ventricular geometry (LV hypertrophy, LV dilatation) • Secondary complications (thrombi, paravalvular leak) • Status of the great vessels.

Tips and Pitfalls

MRI is contraindicated in patients with a prosthetic heart valve whose composition is uncertain • Chest radiographs are often helpful in identifying the valve type.

Selected References

Borger MA et al. Stentless aortic valves are hemodynamically superior to stented valves during mid-term follow-up: a large retrospective study. Ann Thorac Surg 2005; 80: 2180–2185

Hammermeister K et al. Outcomes 15 years after valve replacement with a mechanical versus a bioprosthetic valve: final report of the Veterans Affairs randomized trial. J Am Coll Cardiol 2000; 36: 1152 1158

Jamieson WR. Quantification of haemodynamic performance of stented and stentless aortic bioprostheses and potential influence on survival. Heart Lung Cir 2003; 12: 149–156

Definition

▶ **Epidemiology**
Increasingly popular but technically demanding operation • First performed by Ross in a human patient in 1967 • *Indication:* Isolated aortic valve disease in younger patients (11–50 years of age).

▶ **Etiology, pathophysiology, pathogenesis**
The aortic valve is replaced with the patient's own pulmonary valve • The pulmonary valve is replaced with an aortic or pulmonary allograft (cadaver valve) or bioprosthesis • Very good results are achieved in children and adolescents, because the pulmonary autograft grows with the patient.

Imaging Signs

▶ **Modality of choice**
Echocardiography.

▶ **Echocardiography findings**
Pulmonary valve in the aortic position • Visualization of three pocket-shaped cusps • Potential for aortic insufficiency (possible complication) • Evaluation of RV and LV function and the RVOT • Visualization of the allograft in the pulmonary valve position.

▶ **Chest radiograph and CT findings**
With normal valve function, postoperative images show no cardiopulmonary abnormalities • Allograft or bioprosthesis in the pulmonary valve position • CT is better for evaluating adjacent vascular structures.

▶ **MRI findings**
Same as echocardiography findings • Better delineation of the outflow tracts (RVOT, LVOT) • Analysis of valve function and flow quantification to exclude pulmonary and aortic insufficiency.

▶ **Invasive diagnostic procedures**
Generally not indicated.

Clinical Aspects

▶ **Typical presentation**
Patients with an uncomplicated postoperative course have no clinical problems • Eventual development of aortic insufficiency leads to heart failure.

▶ **Treatment options, course and prognosis**
The Ross operation is the procedure of choice in young adults or patients with a subvalvular abscess.
Advantages. No limitation of physical activities or life style • Excellent long-term function • No need for anticoagulation • Low incidence of thromboembolic complications • Excellent hemodynamics.

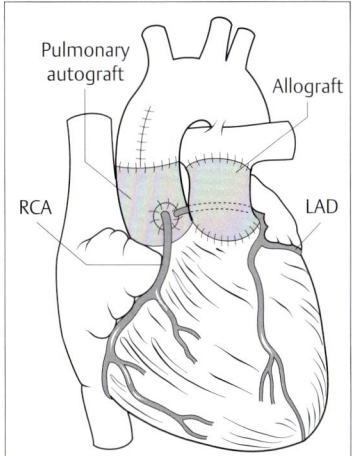

Fig. 3.24 Principle of the Ross operation. The diseased aortic valve is replaced with the patient's own pulmonary valve. The pulmonary valve is replaced with an aortic or pulmonary allograft or bioprosthesis.

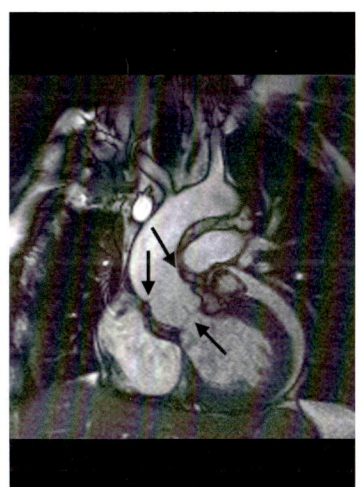

Fig. 3.25 Ross operation in a 55-year-old man. SSFP image in the plane of the LVOT demonstrates the anastomosis and closed pulmonary valve in the aortic position (arrows). Mild postoperative pericardial effusion is noted as an incidental finding (with kind permission of B. Djavidani, University of Regensburg).

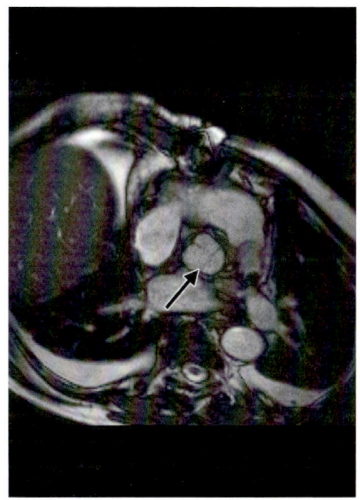

Fig. 3.26 Ross operation in a 55-year-old man. SSFP image parallel to the valve plane demonstrates the closed valve and thin valve cusps (arrow) during diastole. Bilateral pleural effusions are noted as an incidental finding (with kind permission of B. Djavidani, University of Regensburg).

Disadvantages. Technically demanding operation • Significant early mortality • Aortic insufficiency may develop at a later date, necessitating reoperation (up to 15%) • 20-year survival rate 80% • Technically difficult reoperation • Limited availability of allografts.

▶ **What does the clinician want to know?**
Signs of valvular dysfunction • Ventricular function • Pulmonary insufficiency • Right heart dilatation.

Differential Diagnosis

Aortic valve replacement   – Replacement with a mechanical or biologic valve

Tips and Pitfalls

Worldwide hospital mortality is approximately 2.5%, underscoring the need for intensive monitoring during the early postoperative period.

Selected References

Muresian H. The Ross procedure: new insights into the surgical anatomy. Ann Thorac Surg 2006; 81: 495–501

Schmidtke C et al. Up to seven years of experience with the Ross procedure in patients > 60 years of age. J Am Coll Cardiol 2000; 36: 1173–1177

Definition

▶ **Epidemiology**
Technique used rarely during a David reconstruction of the aortic root or a Yacoub replacement of the ascending aorta • Comprises 1% of all aortic valve operations • Used mainly in patients with aortic root aneurysms > 5 cm and/or a type A dissection.

▶ **Etiology, pathophysiology, pathogenesis**
Aneurysms of the aortic root lead to dilatation of the valvular ring and aortic regurgitation • It is generally possible to reconstruct the aortic valve by decalcification, commissurotomy, ring plication, leaflet plication, or valve extension for other indications.

Imaging Signs

▶ **Modality of choice**
Echocardiography.

▶ **Echocardiography findings**
Valve often appears morphologically normal • Mild to moderate residual insufficiency (color Doppler) • Semiquantitative evaluation of the severity of aortic insufficiency • LV dilatation with normal EF • Often these changes normalize through postoperative remodeling.

▶ **Chest radiograph findings**
Sternal cerclage wires after thoracotomy • Other postoperative changes may be seen • Enlarged left cardiac silhouette due to LV dilatation.

▶ **CT findings**
Same findings as on chest radiograph • Detailed visualization of the ascending aorta or a prosthesis following aortic replacement • Reimplanted coronary arteries can be evaluated more accurately by ECG-synchronized multidetector CT.

▶ **MRI findings**
Same morphologic findings as CT • MRI is an excellent follow-up modality • Quantification of LV function (EDV, EF) and regurgitant fraction (flow measurement by phase-velocity mapping).

▶ **Invasive diagnostic procedures**
Patients over 45 years of age should undergo coronary angiography to exclude CHD.

Clinical Aspects

▶ **Typical presentation**
Patients are asymptomatic following an adequate reconstruction.

▶ **Treatment options**
Procedure of choice for isolated aortic valve disease in children and adolescents • Also recommended for aortic root aneurysms (e.g., Marfan syndrome, cystic medial necrosis).

Fig. 3.27 a, b Aortic valve reconstruction in a 62-year-old man with aortic insufficiency secondary to an aortic root aneurysm. SSFP images in the plane of the LVOT. Preoperative image shows marked diastolic regurgitation through the aortic valve (arrow) in the presence of an aortic root aneurysm (**a**). Image taken after prosthetic replacement of the ascending aorta and reimplantation of the coronary arteries (arrow = left coronary artery) shows normal valve closure (**b**). Marked pericardial effusion (small arrows) is still present in the early postoperative period.

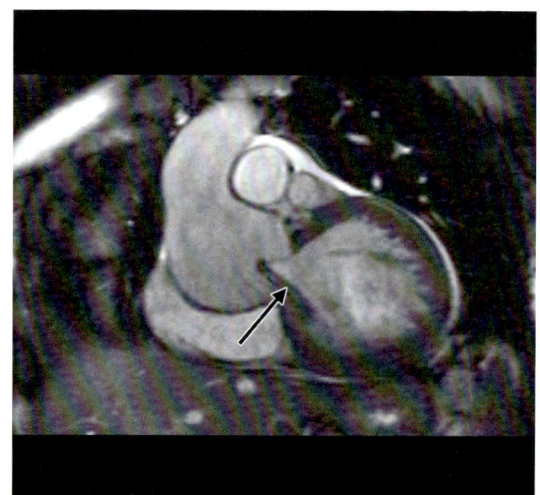

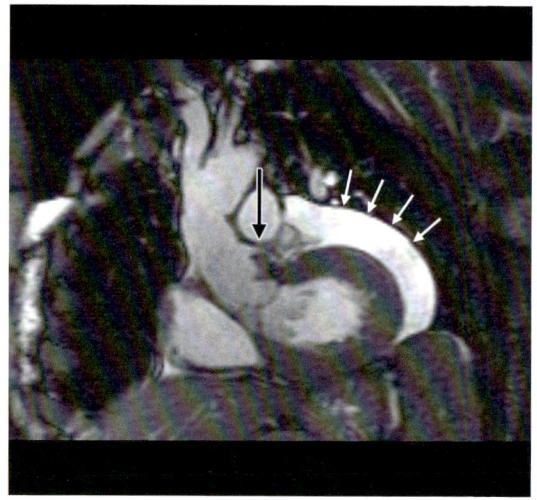

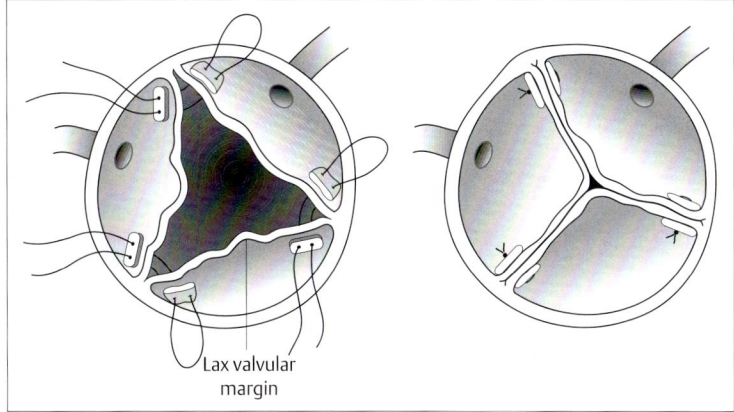

Fig. 3.28 Schematic illustration of an aortic valve reconstruction. Lateral plication sutures are placed in the commissures to tighten the lax leaflet margins. This procedure can eliminate aortic regurgitation while preserving the original valve apparatus.

▶ **Course and prognosis**
Good prognosis in the absence of secondary complications • Endocarditis prophylaxis is required • Low reoperation rate (approximately 0.5–2% at 5 years) • More than 80% rate of patients with grade II aortic insufficiency.

▶ **What does the clinician want to know?**
Persistent aortic insufficiency • LV dilatation • LV function (EF) • Myocardial hypertrophy • Dilatation of the ascending aorta.

Differential Diagnosis

Biologic aortic valve replacement   – Stented or stentless bioprosthesis

Tips and Pitfalls

An adequate reconstruction should be immediately documented by intraoperative TEE.

Selected References

Alsoufi B et al. Results of valve preservation and repair for bicuspid aortic valve insufficiency. J Heart Valve Dis 2005; 14: 752–758
Lausberg HF et al. Valve repair in aortic regurgitation without root dilatation – aortic valve repair. Thorac Cardiovasc Surg 2006; 54: 15–20

Definition

▶ **Epidemiology, etiology**

Most common form of cardiomyopathy (approximately 50%) • Leading cause of heart failure in young adults, with an estimated incidence of 36:100 000 in that population • Primary DCM often has an unknown etiology • Genetic (familial) disposition in up to 35% of cases • Secondary cardiomyopathies often present as DCM.

▶ **Pathoanatomy**

Dilatation of one or both ventricles • Possible involvement of the atria • Myocardial mass is increased, but the wall thickness may appear subjectively normal or decreased.

Imaging Signs

▶ **Modality of choice**

Echocardiography • MRI is the most accurate modality for evaluating morphology and contrast characteristics.

▶ **Chest radiograph and CT findings**

Global enlargement of the heart • Possible dilatation of the pulmonary vessels • Pleural effusion may be present, depending on compensatory status.

▶ **Echocardiographic findings**

Impaired systolic function and dilatation of one or both ventricles.

▶ **MRI findings**

In some cases, MRI may show a typical patchy or linear enhancement pattern (delayed enhancement) that differs from the segmental distribution pattern of myocardial infarction.

▶ **Invasive diagnostic procedures**

Coronary angiography is often necessary to exclude CHD.

Clinical Aspects

▶ **Typical presentation**

All classes of heart failure • Exertional dyspnea • Cardiac arrhythmias.

▶ **Treatment options**

Medical stabilization of heart failure • Cases with LBBB may require cardiac re-synchronization therapy • ICD • Heart transplantation is an option for advanced heart failure.

▶ **Course and prognosis**

Progressive heart failure • Frequent progression to NYHA class III–IV by the time of diagnosis • Sudden cardiac death from arrhythmia.

▶ **What does the clinician want to know?**

Differentiation from other cardiomyopathies and three-vessel CHD • Morphologic and functional status (myocardial mass, ventricular volumes, EF).

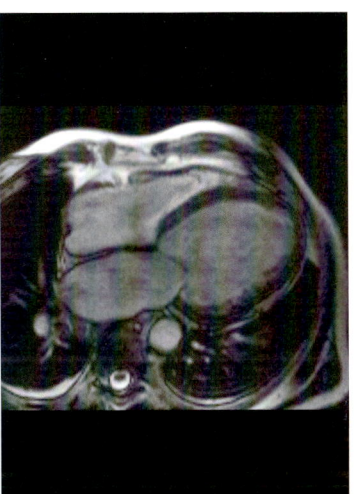

Fig. 4.1   DCM in a 72-year-old man. SSFP image in the four-chamber view shows cardiomegaly with predominant LV dilatation. Mild pleural effusions and dilated pulmonary veins are consistent with chronic congestive heart failure.

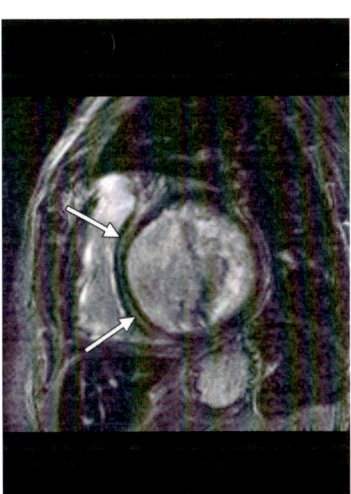

Fig. 4.2   Same patient as in Fig. 4.1. Contrast-enhanced IR GE sequence 15 min after 0.2 mmol gadolinium-DTPA/kg. Short-axis view shows a linear hyperintense area in the septum (arrows) consistent with regional fibrosis.

Differential Diagnosis

Differentiation from other cardiomyopathies	– Morphology – Contrast characteristics (e.g., fatty dysplasia in ARVD, inflammatory infiltrates in myocarditis, sarcoidosis, myocardial hypertrophy in HCM, decreased signal intensity in hemochromatosis)
Differentiation from advanced CHD	– Coronary status (three-vessel disease?) – Contrast characteristics
Differentiation of primary from secondary DCM	– History – Other diseases (toxic cardiomyopathy, myocarditis)

Tips and Pitfalls

The clinical presentation of primary (genetically linked) DCM coincides with that of multivessel CHD, the end stage of toxic injuries (chemotherapeutic agents, alcohol), and previous (viral) myocarditis • Imaging studies can be interpreted only within the context of other parameters (prior history, laboratory findings, coronary status, etc.).

Selected References

Dec GW, Fuster V. Idiopathic dilated cardiomyopathy. New Engl J Med 1994; 331: 1564–1575

McCrohon JA et al. Differentiation of heart failure related to dilated cardiomyopathy and coronary artery disease using gadolinium-enhanced cardiovascular magnetic resonance. Circulation 2003; 108: 54–59

Definition

▶ **Epidemiology**
Present in approximately 1:5000 young adults ● Genetically determined ● Predominantly autosomal dominant mode of inheritance ● Structural changes in the contractile apparatus ● Disturbance of myocyte energy metabolism.

▶ **Pathoanatomy**
Myocardial hypertrophy of one or both ventricles (RV in 30%) ● Often asymmetric (e.g., anteroseptal in approximately 70%) ● HOCM with narrowing of the LVOT in 25% ● Late stage presents morphologic features of DCM (10%).

Imaging Signs

▶ **Modality of choice**
Echocardiography is always the primary study ● May be followed by MRI as a reference study.

▶ **Chest radiograph findings**
Nonspecific findings ● Possible indirect signs of myocardial hypertrophy (raised and rounded left cardiac border) ● Advanced disease presents an enlarged cardiac silhouette and signs of heart failure.

▶ **Echocardiography, MRI, (and CT) findings**
Myocardial hypertrophy ● Possible impairment of systolic and diastolic function ● HOCM leads to systolic anterior motion of the mitral valve through a Venturi effect.

▶ **MRI findings**
Nonsegmental, focal enhancement pattern (delayed enhancement) of the myocardium.

Clinical Aspects

▶ **Typical presentation**
Nonspecific and commonly asymptomatic (incidental finding) ● Dyspnea ● Palpitations (arrhythmias) ● Syncope ● Lethargy ● Angina pectoris, even at rest.

▶ **Treatment options**
Medical stabilization of heart failure ● With HOCM, surgical resection or catheter-assisted embolization of septal coronary branches ● Cardiac pacemaker ● Heart transplantation.

▶ **Course and prognosis**
Leading cause of sudden cardiac death in young adults (usually during exercise) ● Estimated annual mortality is 1% ● Increased risk of myocardial hypertrophy > 30 mm, positive family history, prior history of syncope, asystole, or ventricular tachycardia.

▶ **What does the clinician want to know?**
Quantification of myocardial hypertrophy and ventricular function ● Obstruction of the LVOT ● Contrast characteristics (MRI) ● Differentiation from other diseases.

Fig. 4.3 HCM. SSFP image in the four-chamber view shows myocardial hypertrophy of both ventricles (LV > 12 mm, RV > 3 mm).

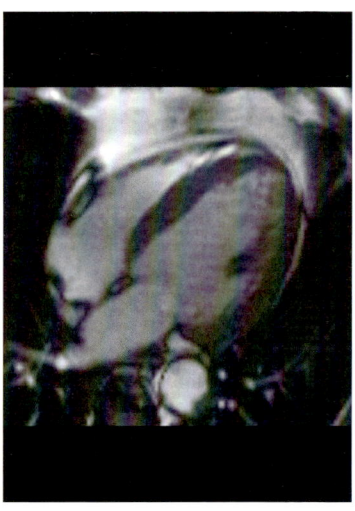

Fig. 4.4 Same patient as in Fig. 4.**3**. Contrast-enhanced IR GE sequence 15 min after 0.2 mmol gadolinium-DTPA/ kg. Short-axis view shows a hyperintense area in the septum (arrow) consistent with regional fibrosis.

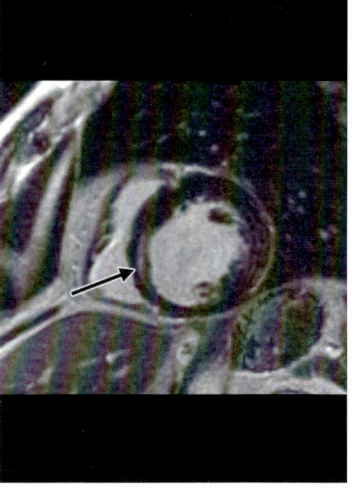

Differential Diagnosis

Other cardiomyopathies associated with myocardial hypertrophy	– E.g., in amyloidosis, hemochromatosis, and uremia (see also RCM)
Other causes of myocardial hypertrophy	– Aortic stenosis
	– Arterial hypertension
	– Athlete's heart (characterized by little to moderate hypertrophy)

Tips and Pitfalls

Consider the clinical information and history when formulating a DD.

Selected References

Fattori R et al. Contribution of magnetic resonance imaging in the differential diagnosis of cardiac amyloidosis and symmetric hypertrophic cardiomyopathy. Am Heart J 1998; 136: 824–830

Moon JC et al. The histologic basis of late gadolinium enhancement cardiovascular magnetic resonance in hypertrophic cardiomyopathy. J Am Coll Cardiol 2004; 43: 2260–2264

Definition

▶ **Epidemiology**
Estimated prevalence of 1:5000 in young adults (< 30 years) • More common in males than in females (2.7:1) • Sporadic occurrence • Some cases show a familial incidence with autosomal dominant transmission • Widely distributed in the Mediterranean region • Mutation in genes that encode desmosomal proteins.

▶ **Pathoanatomy**
RV dilatation with fatty or connective-tissue dysplasia of the myocardium (gross or microscopic) • Reduction in wall thickness • Aneurysms • Trabecular hypertrophy • Possible involvement of the LV (rare).

Imaging Signs

▶ **Modality of choice**
Diagnosis is multimodal based on major and minor criteria (see Chapter 12 [Appendix]) • Echocardiography, ECG, and myocardial biopsy are useful studies • MRI has an important role.

▶ **Echocardiographic and MRI findings**
RV dilatation • Reduction in wall thickness • Akinesia or dyskinesia of circumscribed wall areas (= "bulging") • RV aneurysms • Trabecular hypertrophy (also a criterion in RV ventriculography).

▶ **MRI**
Fatty dysplasia appears as a hyperintense area on T1-weighted images (subepicardial, predominantly on the lateral wall and anterior RVOT) • Connective-tissue dysplasia may appear hyperintense after gadolinium administration.

Clinical Aspects

▶ **Typical presentation**
Arrhythmia, syncope, and sudden cardiac death due to VT (often occurs in young men or athletes during exercise) • In the advanced stage there are signs of right-sided heart failure.

▶ **Treatment options**
Medical treatment for heart failure and arrhythmias • Possible radiofrequency ablation • ICD • Heart transplantation for advanced (biventricular) heart failure.

▶ **Course and prognosis**
Annual mortality is 1–3% • Prognosis better than in VT due to left-sided heart failure.

▶ **What does the clinician want to know?**
RV and LV morphology • Evidence of fatty or connective-tissue dysplasia • Functional abnormalities mainly affect the RV.

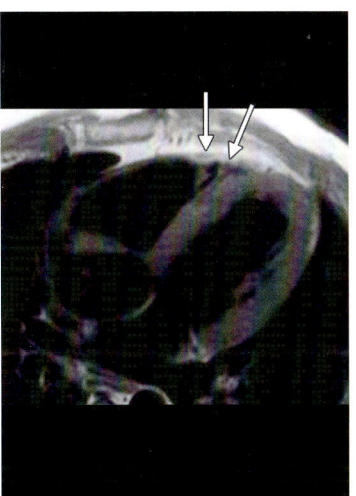

Fig. 4.5 Biopsy-confirmed ARVC in a 30-year-old man. T1-weighted dark-blood FSE sequence in the four-chamber view shows fatty dysplasia of the right ventricular wall, particularly at the insertion of the moderator band (arrows).

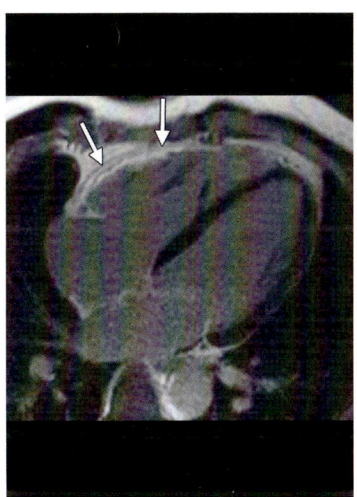

Fig. 4.6 A 38-year-old man with RV tachycardia diagnosed on ECG. IR GE sequence 15 min after 0.2 mmol gadolinium-DTPA/kg demonstrates contrast enhancement in the RV wall (arrows).

Cardiomyopathy

Differential Diagnosis

Other causes of arrhythmias or VT	– Idiopathic RV tachycardia without ARVC
	– Other cardiomyopathies
	– Peri- or myocarditis
	– CHD
Congenital disorders	– Uhl's disease (RV hypoplasia)
	– ASD
	– VSD

Tips and Pitfalls

Negative imaging findings do not rule out ARVC! ● Always consider other causes due to the overlap with other diseases, e.g., fatty myocardial degeneration and cardiac arrhythmias may also result from myocarditis or infarction.

Selected References

Basso C et al. Arrhythmogenic right ventricular cardiomyopathy: Dysplasia, dystrophy or myocarditis? Circulation 1996; 94: 983–991

Castillo E et al. Arrhythmogenic right ventricular dysplasia: ex vivo and in vivo fat detection with black-blood MR imaging. Radiology 2004; 232: 38–48

Definition

▶ **Epidemiology**
Very rare in Western countries • Idiopathic cause • More common in tropical countries as endomyocardial fibrosis • Some secondary cardiomyopathies may display features of RCM.

▶ **Etiology, pathophysiology, pathogenesis**
Small ventricles with normal systolic function and impaired diastolic relaxation • High ventricular filling pressures due to endocardial fibrosis • Dilatation of the atria.

Imaging Signs

▶ **Modality of choice**
Echocardiography • MRI is most useful in patients with suspected amyloidosis, sarcoidosis, etc.

▶ **Chest radiograph and CT findings**
Enlargement of the atria • Signs of pulmonary venous congestion • Pleural effusion.

▶ **Echocardiographic and MRI findings**
Impaired ventricular filling • Normal-sized ventricles • Normal systolic function (low EDV, normal EF) • Diastolic dysfunction • Pericardial thickening is a hallmark of the most important differential diagnosis, constrictive pericarditis.

▶ **MRI findings**
Used mainly in patients with suspected secondary cardiomyopathy • Findings in these cases may include altered contrast characteristics and/or T2-weighted signal characteristics due to amyloidosis, sarcoidosis, or hemochromatosis.

Clinical Aspects

▶ **Typical presentation**
Heart failure (dyspnea, lethargy, edema, pleural effusion) • Frequent atrial arrhythmias (atrial fibrillation, AV block) • Syncope and sudden cardiac death due to bradycardic and tachycardic arrhythmias.

▶ **Treatment options**
Medical treatment for heart failure and arrhythmias • Anticoagulation in patients with atrial fibrillation • Patients may need a cardiac pacemaker • Heart transplantation is a last resort.

▶ **Course and prognosis**
Poor prognosis in children • 5-year survival rate of 95% in adults.

▶ **What does the clinician want to know?**
Morphologic criteria • Pericardial thickening • Quantification of ventricular function (MRI) • Myocardial signal and contrast characteristics (MRI) • Differentiation from other conditions.

Fig. 4.7   Postendocarditis endocardial fibrosis in a 52-year-old woman. SSFP image in the four-chamber view shows small ventricles with dilatation of the LA. There is a thrombus on the LV lateral wall with fixation of the chordae tendineae and secondary mitral insufficiency (arrows).

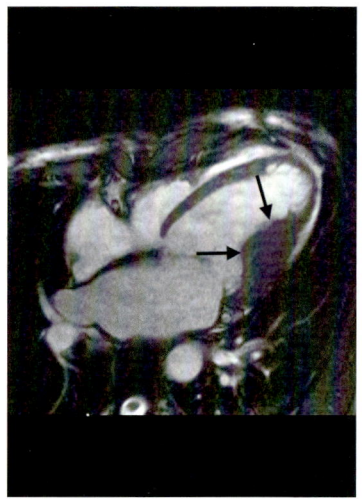

Fig. 4.8   SSFP image in the four-chamber view. The mixed pattern of patchy and nodular pericardial thickening (arrows) is typical of constrictive pericarditis, which is always included in the DD of RCM.

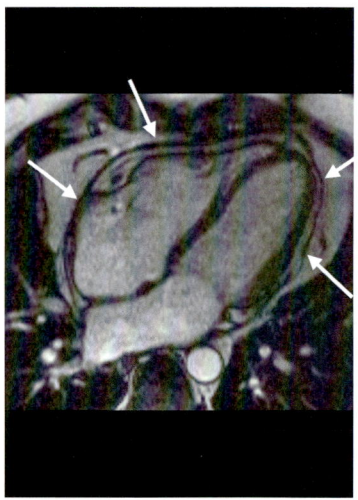

Differential Diagnosis

Secondary cardiomyo-pathies associated with myocardial restriction	– Amyloidosis – Hemochromatosis – Sarcoidosis – Storage diseases – Carcinoid – Systemic diseases (e.g., scleroderma) – History of radiotherapy or chemotherapy – Pericardial metastases
Inflammatory causes	– Löffler endocarditis (hypereosinophilic syndrome) – Tropical endocardial fibrosis (caused by parasites, etc.)

Tips and Pitfalls

Evaluate for secondary cardiomyopathies and other causes of myocardial restriction that should be considered in the DD.

Selected References

Hancock EW. Differenzial diagnosis of restrictive cardiomyopathy and constrictive peri-carditis. Heart 2001; 86: 343–349

Schneider U et al. Long term follow up of patients with endomyocardial fibrosis: effects of surgery. Heart 1998; 79: 362–367

Definition

▶ **Epidemiology**
ILNC is an unclassified cardiomyopathy based on a mutation of the G4.5 gene (encodes the taffazin protein) and characterized by a failure of myocardial compaction during intrauterine development.

▶ **Etiology, pathophysiology, pathogenesis**
Normal-sized or dilated LV with pronounced trabeculation extending into the outer layers of the myocardial wall ● RV may also be affected ● Impaired systolic function.

Imaging Signs

▶ **Modality of choice**
Echocardiography ● MRI.

▶ **Chest radiograph and CT findings**
Normal findings ● Advanced stages may show signs of left-sided heart failure with enlarged cardiac silhouette ● CT can demonstrate the increased trabeculation of the LV.

▶ **Echocardiographic and MRI findings**
Morphologic changes ● Impaired systolic function ● Quantification of functional parameters ● MRI is preferred for evaluating the RV.

Clinical Aspects

▶ **Typical presentation**
Asymptomatic in early life ● Often diagnosed initially in adulthood ● Heart failure ● Tachyarrhythmias ● Sudden cardiac death ● Thromboembolism.

▶ **Treatment options**
Symptomatic treatment of heart failure ● ICD ● Heart transplantation.

▶ **Course and prognosis**
Poor prognosis with annual mortality of 9%.

▶ **What does the clinician want to know?**
Morphologic criteria ● Quantification of ventricular function (echocardiography, MRI) ● Thrombi.

Differential Diagnosis

The differential diagnosis should include DCM and secondary cardiomyopathies that have the same presentation as DCM.

Tips and Pitfalls

In rare cases the disease may be associated with an ASD, VSD, or stenosis of the RVOT (pulmonary stenosis).

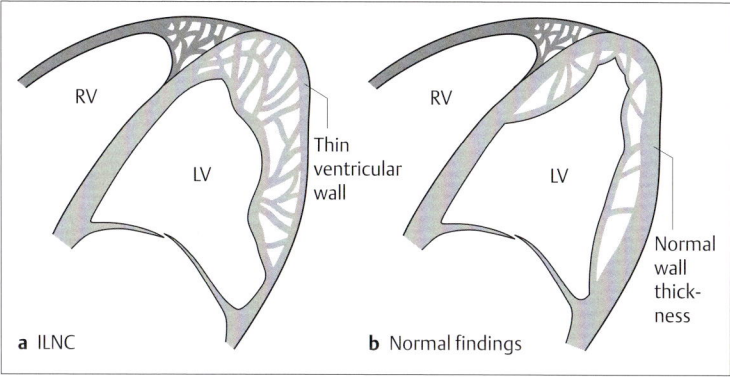

Fig. 4.9 a, b Schematic illustration of ILNC. The trabeculation of the LV myocardium extends into the outer wall layers.

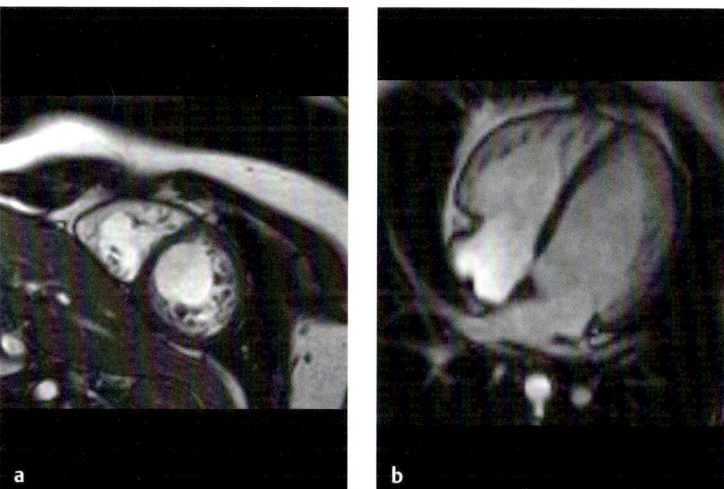

Fig. 4.10 a, b ILNC in a 22-year-old man with recurrent episodes of ventricular tachycardia. Cine-SSFP images in the short-axis and four-chamber views show markedly increased trabeculation of both ventricles.

Selected References

Murphy RT et al. Natural history and familial characteristics of isolated left ventricular non-compaction. Eur Heart J 2005; 26: 187–192

Rigopoulos A et al. Isolated left ventricular noncompaction: an unclassified cardiomyopathy with severe prognosis in adults. Cardiology 2002; 98: 25–32

Definition

▶ **Epidemiology**
Recently described syndrome ● Predominantly affects middle-aged women ● Reversible ● Symptoms resemble myocardial infarction ● Described in Japan as *tako-tsubo* ("octopus trap") cardiomyopathy ● Believed to be precipitated by emotional stress.

▶ **Etiology, pathophysiology, pathogenesis**
Etiology uncertain ● Coronary spasm, microvascular ischemia, and myocarditis have been proposed ● Coronary status and cardiac morphology are normal.

Imaging Signs

▶ **Modality of choice**
Coronary angiography to exclude CHD ● MRI to assess myocardial viability.

▶ **Chest radiograph and CT findings**
Normal findings.

▶ **Echocardiographic and MRI findings**
Typical functional disturbance consisting of apical and inferior hypo- or akinesia (apical ballooning).

▶ **MRI and SPECT findings**
Exclusion of myocardial infarction.

Clinical Aspects

▶ **Typical presentation**
Symptoms of acute myocardial infarction ● Chest pain, angina pectoris ● ST-segment changes ● Slight troponin and CK elevation.

▶ **Treatment options**
Symptomatic treatment same as for heart failure and acute myocardial ischemia.

▶ **Course and prognosis**
Symptoms are always reversible in days to weeks ● Lethal complications have not been described.

▶ **What does the clinician want to know?**
Morphologic changes ● Evidence of myocardial ischemia or infarction or inflammatory changes (edema, pericardial effusion, contrast enhancement).

Differential Diagnosis

Angina pectoris	– CHD
Myocardial infarction	– CHD
Inflammatory heart disease	– Pericarditis
	– Myocarditis

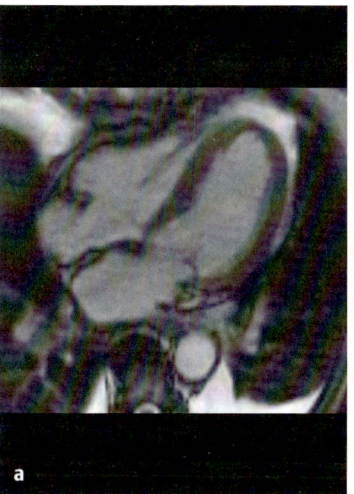 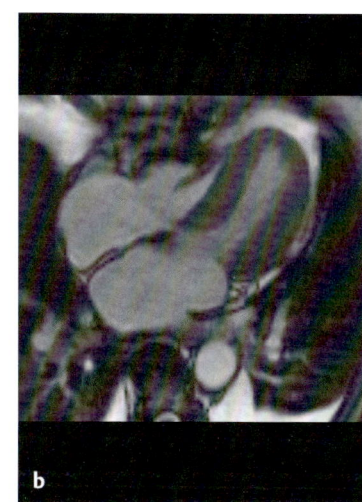

Fig. 4.11 a, b   Apical ballooning syndrome in a 76-year-old woman. Cine-SSFP images in the four-chamber view at end diastole and end systole demonstrate apical dyskinesia with an aneurysm. Bilateral pleural effusions are also present.

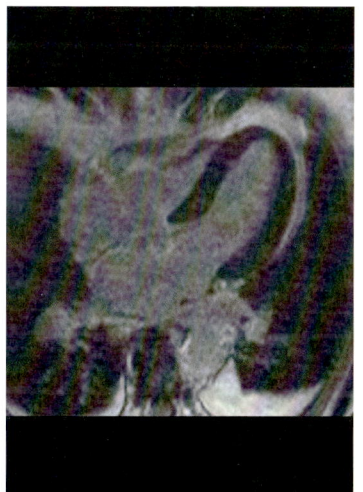

Fig. 4.12   IR GE sequence 15 min after gadolinium-DTPA excludes myocardial infarction. There is no apical contrast enhancement of the LV.

Tips and Pitfalls

Coronary stenosis should always be excluded by coronary angiography.

Selected References

Kuriso S et al. Tako-tsubo-like left ventricular dysfunction with ST-segment elevation: A novel cardiac syndrome mimicking acute myocardial infarction. Am Heart J 2002; 243: 448–455

Sharkey SW et al. Acute and reversible cardiomyopathy provoked by stress in women from the United States. Circulation 2005; 111: 472–479

Definition

▶ **Epidemiology**
Systemic granulomatous disease • Sites of predilection are the hilar lymph nodes, lung (90%), eyes, and skin • All organ systems may be affected • Cardiac involvement is present in approximately 25% of cases by autopsy (perhaps more often).

▶ **Etiology, pathophysiology, pathogenesis**
Two patterns of cardiac involvement are distinguished:
– Focal involvement by noncaseating epithelioid cell granulomas.
– Diffuse granulomatous infiltration.
Sites of predilection in the heart are the septum, posterior wall, and conduction system (particularly the AV node).

Imaging Signs

▶ **Modality of choice**
MRI.

▶ **Chest radiograph and CT findings**
Stage-dependent • Hilar lymphadenopathy and/or pulmonary involvement • Involvement of other organ systems.

▶ **Echocardiographic findings**
Regional myocardial thickening (hyperechoic) • Hypokinesia (granulomas).

▶ **MRI findings**
Granulomas have high T2-weighted signal intensity and show gadolinium enhancement • Cases with diffuse involvement may show only global impairment of ventricular function.

▶ **Nuclear medicine**
May be useful in selected patients with suspected CHD • Perfusion defects regress during exercise.

▶ **Invasive diagnostic procedures**
Coronary angiography can be used in selected cases to exclude CHD • Myocardial biopsy often yields false-negative results.

Clinical Aspects

▶ **Typical presentation**
Systemic manifestations of sarcoidosis in one-third of patients (night sweats, fever, lethargy, weight loss) • Rhythm disorders (AV block, arrhythmias) • Sudden cardiac death • Heart failure.

▶ **Treatment options**
Corticosteroids • Other immunosuppressants • Cardiac pacemaker • ICD.

▶ **Course and prognosis**
Life expectancy ranges from 2 to more than 10 years, depending on the overall course.

Fig. 4.13 Cardiac sarcoidosis in a 28-year-old man. SSFP sequence reveals nodular thickening of the inferior wall (arrow).

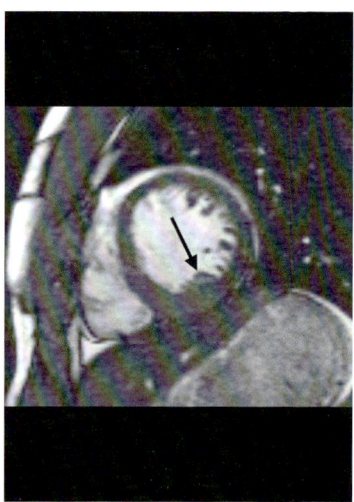

Fig. 4.14 IR GE sequence after gadolinium-DTPA administration in the same patient shows enhancement of the morphologically suspicious area based on granulomatous myocardial infiltration (arrow).

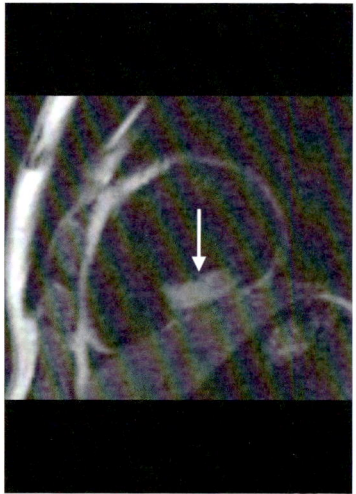

▶ **What does the clinician want to know?**
Evidence of cardiac involvement (detectable granulomas: high T2-weighted signal intensity, enhance after gadolinium administration) • Myocardial morphology and function.

Differential Diagnosis

Other causes of arrhythmias and heart failure	– Idiopathic arrhythmias, CHD, other cardiomyopathies

Tips and Pitfalls

Diffuse involvement is difficult to diagnose even with MRI • Arrhythmias and ventricular dysfunction may be the only evidence of diffuse disease.

Selected References

Shimada T et al. Diagnosis of cardiac sarcoidosis and evaluation of the effects of steroid therapy by gadolinium-DTPA enhanced magnetic resonance imaging. Am J Med 2001; 110: 520–527

Uemura A et al. Histologic diagnostic rate of cardiac sarcoidosis: evaluation of endomyocardial biopsies. Am Heart J 1999; 138: 299–302

Definition

▶ **Epidemiology**
Three forms are distinguished:
- *Primary amyloidosis:* Myocardial involvement in 50%.
- *Secondary amyloidosis:* E.g., in plasmacytoma, rheumatoid arthritis, or inflammatory bowel disease; cardiac involvement in 10%.
- *Hereditary amyloidosis:* Autosomal dominant mode of inheritance, cardiac involvement in 5%.

▶ **Etiology, pathophysiology, pathogenesis**
Amyloid deposits in the interstitial space of the myocardium and coronary arteries ● Results in mural hypertrophy and coronary stenoses (especially of the small coronary arteries) ● The myocardium has a rubbery consistency, with a restricting effect ● Systolic function is initially normal.

Imaging Signs

▶ **Modality of choice**
MRI.

▶ **Chest radiograph and CT findings**
Obliteration or widening of the cardiac silhouette indicating pericardial effusion ● Pleural effusion ● Possible pulmonary involvement.

▶ **Echocardiographic findings**
Myocardial thickening with inhomogeneous hyperechoic pattern ● Impaired diastolic function ● Pericardial effusion.

▶ **MRI findings**
Impaired diastolic function ● Enhancing area with inhomogeneous high T2 signal intensity ● Pericardial and pleural effusion ● Possible pulmonary involvement.

▶ **Myocardial nuclear medicine findings**
May be useful in selected patients with suspected CHD ● Perfusion defects *regress* during exercise.

▶ **Invasive diagnostic procedures**
Histologic confirmation of initial organ involvement at other sites such as the rectum (80%), bone marrow (50%), and skin (50–90%) ● Myocardial biopsy may be considered in exceptional cases.

Clinical Aspects

▶ **Typical presentation**
Heart failure ● Syncope ● Arrhythmias ● Pericardial effusion.

▶ **Treatment options**
Chemotherapy ● High-dose chemotherapy with stem-cell transplantation.

▶ **Course and prognosis**
Very poor prognosis ● Average life expectancy is 1 year.

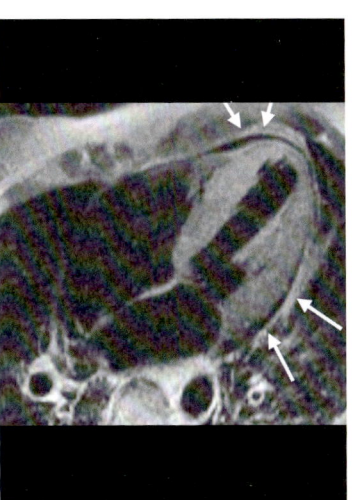

Fig. 4.15 Plasmacytoma and cardiac amyloidosis in a 60-year-old woman. Fat-saturated T1-weighted dark-blood TSE sequence. Four-chamber view shows pronounced myocardial hypertrophy in all wall segments. The arrows indicate distention of the pericardial layers due to pericardial effusion.

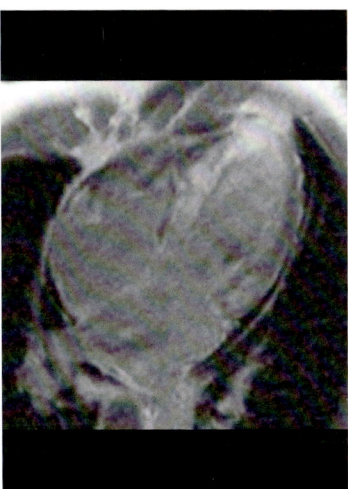

Fig. 4.16 IR GE sequence after gadolinium-DTPA administration. Four-chamber view shows diffuse enhancement of all wall segments.

▶ **What does the clinician want to know?**
Myocardial thickening ● Signs of amyloid deposits on T2-weighted image or after contrast administration (MRI) ● Functional parameters, signs of restriction ● Pericardial effusion.

Differential Diagnosis

RCM, HCM, CHD ● In the presence of confirmed amyloidosis and the occurrence of new cardiac symptoms, there should be a high index of suspicion for myocardial involvement.

Tips and Pitfalls

Normal MRI findings do not exclude early-stage cardiac amyloidosis.

Selected References

Fattori R et al. Contribution of magnetic resonance imaging in the differential diagnosis of cardiac amyloidosis and symmetric hypertrophic cardiomyopathy. Am Heart J 1998; 136: 824–830

Maceira AM et al. Cardiovascular magnetic resonance in cardiac amyloidosis. Circulation 2005; 111: 186–193

Definition

▶ **Etiology**
- *Primary hemochromatosis:* Impairment of iron uptake • Autosomal recessive mode of inheritance.
- *Secondary hemochromatosis, hemosiderosis:* Causes include repeated blood transfusions over a period of years (aplastic or sickle cell anemia, thalassemia) • Cardiac involvement in up to 86% of cases.

▶ **Etiology, pathophysiology, pathogenesis**
Progressive deposition of iron in myocardial cells • Late stage is marked by displacement of myofibrils • Cellular degeneration and fibrosis • Gross cardiac enlargement and hypertrophy.

Imaging Signs

▶ **Modality of choice**
MRI.

▶ **Chest radiograph findings**
Often normal • May show enlarged cardiac silhouette • Possible signs of heart failure (pulmonary venous congestion, pleural effusion).

▶ **CT findings**
Same as chest radiograph findings • Demonstrates myocardial hypertrophy.

▶ **Echocardiographic and MRI findings**
RV and LV dilatation • Myocardial hypertrophy • Impaired systolic and diastolic function • Possible increase in myocardial echogenicity.
MRI shows decreased myocardial signal intensity in T1-, T2-, and T2*-weighted sequences • T2*-weighted signal intensity correlates closely with myocardial iron content and is useful for monitoring response to chelation therapy.

▶ **Invasive diagnostic procedures**
Confirmation by myocardial biopsy is necessary only in extremely rare cases.

Clinical Aspects

▶ **Typical presentation**
Elevated hepatic enzymes • Hepatomegaly • Arthropathy • Heart failure that increases with myocardial iron content • Cardiac arrhythmias may occur.

▶ **Treatment options**
Chelation therapy.

▶ **Course and prognosis**
Iron deposits should clear in response to chelation therapy • Rate of cardiac deaths in thalassemia major is 71%.

▶ **What does the clinician want to know?**
Morphologic and functional status of the heart • Evidence of iron deposits (MRI: T2- and/or T2*-weighted images).

Fig. 4.17 Cardiac involvement in hemochromatosis in a 53-year-old man. T2-weighted FSE image in the four-chamber view shows predominantly septal myocardial hypertrophy.

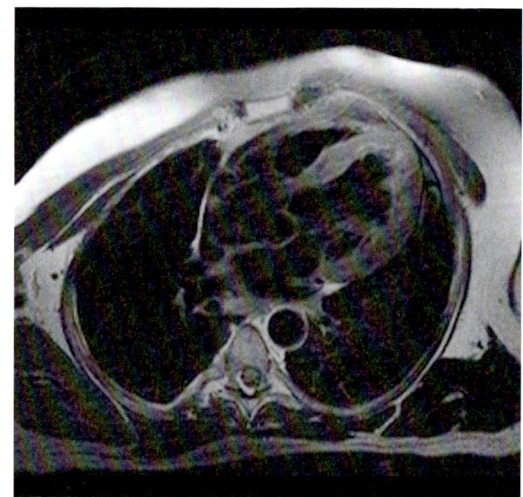

Fig. 4.18 Same patient as in Fig. 4.**17**. SSFP image in the short-axis view shows predominantly inferoseptal myocardial thickening.

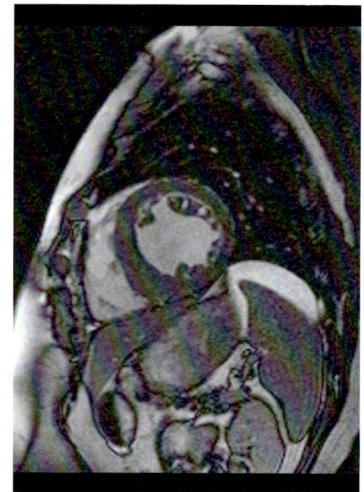

Differential Diagnosis

Cardiac involvement in hemochromatosis presents mixed features of RCM and DCM. It should therefore be considered in the DD of patients with corresponding unexplained complaints.

Tips and Pitfalls

Cardiac involvement in hemochromatosis is more common than expected and may occur independently of other commonly affected organs (liver, spleen, skin, pancreas, etc.).

Selected References

Cohen AR et al. Thalassemia. Hematology; 2004; 14–34

Ptaszek LM et al. Early diagnosis of hemochromatosis-related cardiomyopathy with magnetic resonance imaging. J Cardiovasc Magn Reson. 2005; 7: 689–692

Definition

▶ **Epidemiology**
Develops in up to 80% of patients with end-stage renal failure on hemodialysis or after renal transplantation.

▶ **Etiology, pathophysiology, pathogenesis**
Multifactorial etiology ● Besides unknown causes, the main established causes are anemia, arterial hypertension, hypervolemia, and metabolic factors (uremia) ● Cardiac dilatation and hypertrophy ● Myocardial fibrosis ● Atherosclerotic changes in all vessels including the coronary arteries and heart valves.

Imaging Signs

▶ **Modality of choice**
Echocardiography (should be used for early monitoring).

▶ **Chest radiograph and CT findings**
Advanced stages show signs of hypervolemia and heart failure ● Myocardial hypertrophy (rounded and elevated left cardiac border) ● Calcifications of vessels, heart valves, and pericardium (uremic pericarditis).

▶ **Echocardiographic and MRI findings**
LV dilatation ● Myocardial hypertrophy ● Impaired systolic and diastolic function ● Pericardial effusion ● Thickening and dysfunction of the mitral and aortic valves (increased incidence of aortic stenosis) ● MRI may show focal delayed enhancement after gadolinium administration.

▶ **Invasive diagnostic procedures**
Coronary angiography is indicated in patients with suspected CHD.

Clinical Aspects

▶ **Typical presentation**
Progression of heart failure and cardiac arrhythmias over time ● Aortic stenosis ● Syncopal episodes ● Angina pectoris in patients with CHD.

▶ **Treatment options**
Appropriate treatment for hypertension and anemia ● Optimized dialysis regimen ● Correction of metabolic disorders.

▶ **Course and prognosis**
Cardiac complications (cardiomyopathy and CHD) determine the prognosis ● The 10-year survival rate is approximately 50%.

▶ **What does the clinician want to know?**
Myocardial hypertrophy ● Functional status of cardiac valves and ventricles ● Pericardial changes ● CHD.

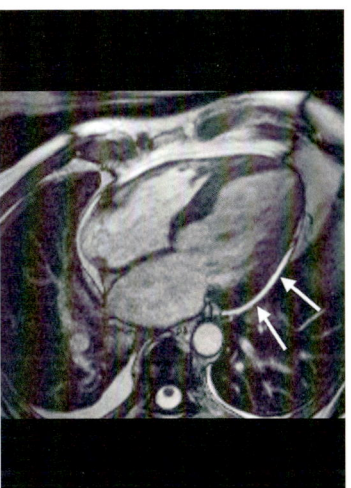

Fig. 4.19 End-stage renal failure in a 62-year-old man on hemodialysis. SSFP image in the four-chamber view (end diastole) shows dilatation of the LV and LA and myocardial hypertrophy. Pleural effusions and a mild pericardial effusion (arrows) are also present.

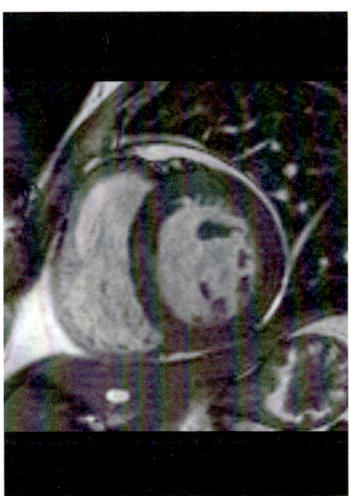

Fig. 4.20 Same patient as in Fig. 4.**19**. SSFP image in the short-axis view shows predominantly septal hypertrophy to 18 mm (septum).

Differential Diagnosis

Myocardial hypertrophy due to arterial hypertension	– Usually a known history of hypertension
Myocardial hypertrophy due to aortic stenosis	– Aortic configuration of the cardiac silhouette – Calcification and fibrosis of the aortic valve with restricted opening

Tips and Pitfalls

Always consider the possibility of uremic cardiomyopathy and (asymptomatic) CHD in dialysis patients. Postinfarction scars (delayed enhancement) may be detected incidentally on postgadolinium MRI.

Selected References

Kunz K et al. Uremic cardiomyopathy. Nephrol Dial Transplant 1998; 13 (Supp 4): 39–43
Mark PB et al. Redefinition of uremic cardiomyopathy by contrast-enhanced cardiac magnetic resonance imaging. Kidney Int 2006; 69: 1839–1845

Definition

▶ **Etiology**
Direct injury of the endocardium, myocardium, or pericardium by toxic compounds (e.g., anthracyclines, alkylating agents, antimetabolites, alcohol).

▶ **Epidemiology**
Many cases are dose dependent (e.g., total dose of more than 550 mg/m^2 doxorubicin or 80 g alcohol/day for 10 years) • Toxic cardiomyopathy is classified as acute (hours to days), chronic (1–12 months, most common form), or late (occurring years later).

▶ **Etiology, pathophysiology, pathogenesis**
Pathogenic mechanisms are direct cell denaturation (alcohol) or formation of free radicals (anthracyclines) • Most cases present clinically with the picture of DCM • Myocardial hypertrophy may occur • Histologic changes consist of vacuolar myocardial degeneration, loss of myofibrils, and interstitial fibrosis.

Imaging Signs

▶ **Modality of choice**
Echocardiography (for early monitoring).

▶ **Chest radiograph and CT findings**
Often normal • May show enlarged cardiac silhouette • Heart failure (pericardial and pleural effusion).

▶ **Echocardiographic and MRI findings**
RV and LV dilatation • Possible myocardial hypertrophy • Impaired systolic and diastolic function • Pericardial effusion • MRI may show areas of pericardial thickening or fibrosis • Delayed enhancement after contrast administration.

▶ **Invasive diagnostic procedures**
Generally not required • Some authors have suggested that invasive tests have prognostic value in the anthracycline-induced form.

Clinical Aspects

▶ **Typical presentation**
Heart failure • Paroxysmal atrial fibrillation (alcohol) • Tachycardic arrhythmias.

▶ **Treatment options**
Symptomatic treatment of heart failure • Abstinence from alcohol • Dose reduction or change to alternative chemotherapeutic agents.

▶ **Course and prognosis**
Findings should improve on withdrawal of the offending agent • The 4-year mortality rate of overt disease is approximately 5–30% in cases caused by anthracyclines and cyclophosphamide, and over 50% in cases caused by chronic alcohol misuse.

▶ **What does the clinician want to know?**
Morphologic and functional status of the heart • Pericardial changes.

Cardiomyopathy

Fig. 4.21 Toxic cardiomyopathy following anthracycline therapy in a 19-year-old man. SSFP image in the four-chamber view demonstrates cardiomegaly and a mild pericardial effusion (arrows).

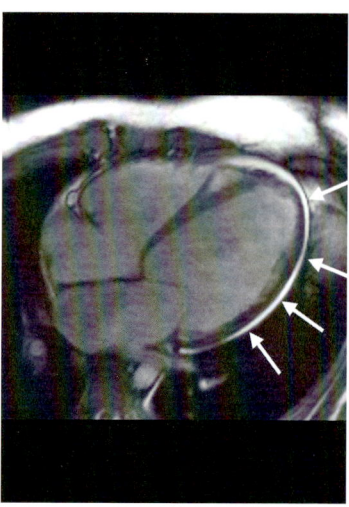

Fig. 4.22 Same patient as in Fig. 4.21. IR GE sequence 15 min after 0.15 mmol gadolinium-DTPA/kg shows enhancement in the basal portion of the lateral myocardial wall (arrow).

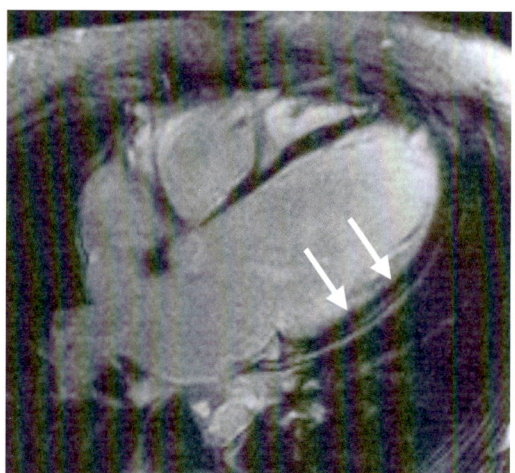

Differential Diagnosis

DCM, HCM, pericarditis.

Tips and Pitfalls

A lack of clinical information and ignorance of the long-term history may prompt the erroneous diagnosis of a primary cardiomyopathy.

Selected References

Edward TH et al. Cardiovascular Complications of Cancer Therapy: Diagnosis, Pathogenesis, and Management. Circulation 2004; 109: 3122–3131

Definition

▶ **Epidemiology**

Inflammatory disease of the myocardium due to various causes • Incidence unknown • The "typical" patient is a young man.

▶ **Etiology, pathophysiology, pathogenesis**

Viruses are the main causative organism, accounting for approximately 50% of cases • Inflammatory infiltration or cell necrosis may occur, depending on the severity of the disease • Initial changes give way to fibrosis and fatty dystrophy • A chronic course may result from persistence of the causative organism or an autoimmune response.

Imaging Signs

▶ **Modality of choice**

Echocardiography • MRI as a second-line method is steadily gaining in importance.

▶ **Chest radiograph and CT findings**

Often normal findings • May demonstrate pericardial effusion • Pulmonary infiltrates and lymphomas in the setting of an infection • Inflammatory cardiomyopathy may produce an enlarged cardiac silhouette.

▶ **Echocardiographic findings**

Normal echocardiography findings are not uncommon • Impaired diastolic function, followed later by impaired systolic function and additional diastolic impairment • Myocardial thickening (edema) • Pericardial effusion in patients with associated pericarditis.

▶ **MRI findings**

Same as echocardiographic findings • Better visualization of the pericardium • Focal increase in T2-weighted signal intensity (edema, granulomatous infiltrates) • Acquisition of postgadolinium images (IR GE sequence) is mandatory.

▶ **SPECT and PET findings**

Examination with antimyosin antibodies can detect myocardial injury with high sensitivity but low specificity.

▶ **Invasive diagnostic procedures**

May be done in the acute stage to exclude an acute coronary syndrome • Myocardial biopsy can establish the diagnosis • *Caution:* high rate of false-negative results.

Clinical Aspects

▶ **Typical presentation**

Often asymptomatic initially • Possible nonspecific signs of viral infection • Heart failure • Cardiac arrhythmia • Chest pain.

▶ **Treatment options**

No specific treatment is available at present • Restriction of physical activity • Symptomatic therapy • Virostatics are under investigation.

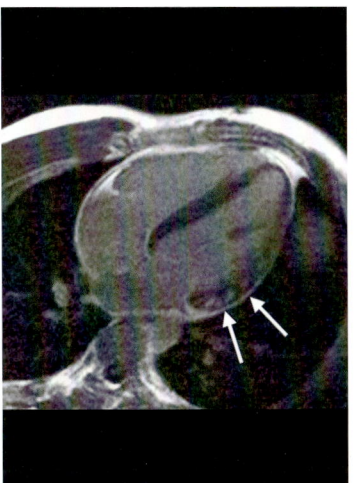

Fig. 5.1 Myocarditis in a 15-year-old boy. IR GE sequence 15 min after administration of 0.2 mmol/kg gadolinium-DTPA/kg. Four-chamber view shows hyperintense areas in the lateral basal wall of the myocardium (arrows), signifying inflammation.

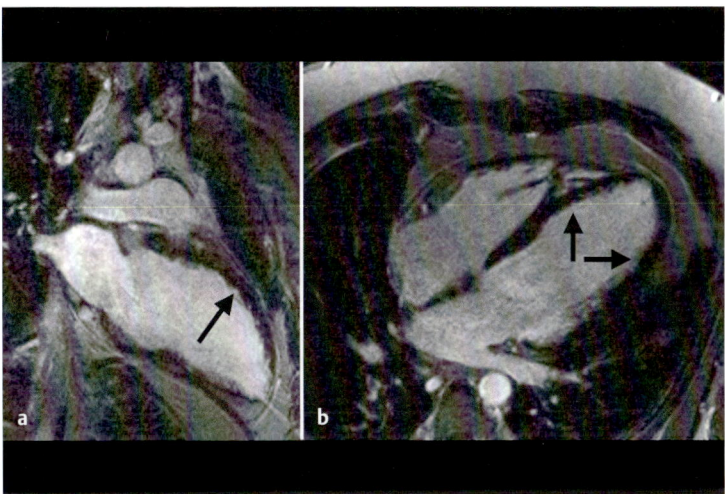

Fig. 5.2 a, b MR image in a 32-year-old man with systemic lupus erythematosus. Contrast-enhanced IR GE sequence 15 min after administration of 0.2 mmol gadolinium-DTPA/kg. Four-chamber and long-axis views at 3 T demonstrate endomyocardial enhancement (arrows).

▶ **Course and prognosis**

Highly variable • Spontaneous resolution is common • May progress to DCM or inflammatory cardiomyopathy, with a possible fatal outcome • Heart failure is considered a poor prognostic sign.

▶ **What does the clinician want to know?**

Signs of heart failure • Extracardiac manifestations • Cardiac function • Pericardial effusion • Inflammatory myocardial and pericardial changes (MRI).

Differential Diagnosis

Cardiac causes	– Acute coronary syndrome
	– Myocardial infarction
	– Pericarditis
Extracardiac causes	– Aortic dissection
	– Pulmonary embolism
Chronic stage	– DCM
	– Inflammatory cardiomyopathy

Tips and Pitfalls

(Peri-)myocarditis should be considered in the differential diagnosis of patients with acute chest pain, normal coronary status, an abnormal ECG, or abnormal levels of enzymes such as CK and troponin.

Selected References

Mahrholdt H et al. Cardiovascular magnetic resonance assessment of human myocarditis: a comparison to histology and molecular pathology. Circulation. 2004; 109: 1250–1258

Definition

▶ **Etiology**
Variety of causes: Infectious ● Autoimmune ● Metabolic ● Toxic ● Neoplastic ● Traumatic ● Idiopathic ● Idiopathic and infectious causes are responsible for approximately 80% of cases.

▶ **Pathophysiology, pathogenesis**
Pericardial thickening and fibrous exudation during the acute phase (audible "pericardial rub," pericarditis sicca) ● Often accompanied by pericardial effusion (exudative pericarditis) ● Myocardial involvement may occur (perimyocarditis) ● Over time, pericarditis may lead to fibrous adhesion of the pericardial layers with regional constriction of the heart ● Late sequelae may include calcifications (constrictive pericarditis).

Imaging Signs

▶ **Modality of choice**
Echocardiography ● MRI provides the highest sensitivity in equivocal cases.

▶ **Chest radiograph and CT findings**
Often normal findings ● May show signs of pericardial effusion ● Pulmonary infiltrates and lymphomas in the setting of infection ● CT may demonstrate pericardial thickening.

▶ **Echocardiographic findings**
Pericardial effusion ● Diastolic dysfunction due to constriction ● Limited ability to evaluate pericardial morphology.

▶ **MRI findings**
Same as Echocardiographic findings ● Better visualization of the pericardium ● Pericardial thickening and effusion ● Contrast-enhanced imaging in acute inflammation (fat-saturated dark-blood T1-weighted TSE or IR GE sequence).

▶ **Invasive testing**
May be appropriate in selected cases to exclude an acute coronary syndrome (see also Postinfarction Pericarditis and Dressler Syndrome).

Clinical Aspects

▶ **Typical presentation**
Systemic inflammatory signs (fever, cough) ● Retrosternal chest pain that improves on sitting up and leaning forward ● ECG changes in 90% of patients ● May take an asymptomatic course (e.g., in collagen diseases or uremia).

▶ **Treatment options**
Steroidal and nonsteroidal anti-inflammatory agents ● Aspirin ● Antibiotics ● Pericardial drainage for hemodynamically significant effusion or pericardial tamponade.

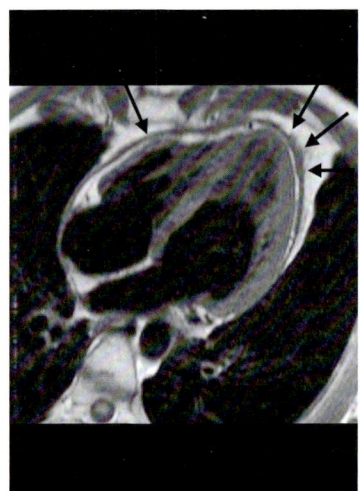 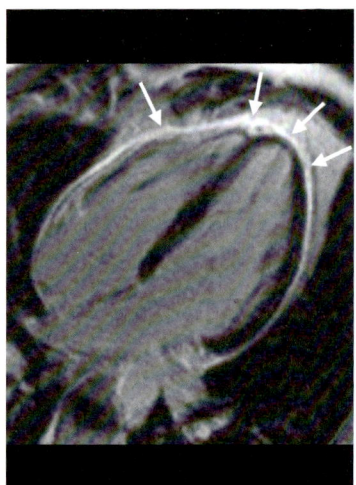

Fig. 5.3 Acute pericarditis in a 37-year-old man. T1-weighted dark-blood TSE sequence in the four-chamber plane shows marked thickening and ill-defined margins of the pericardium (arrows). There is no pericardial effusion!

Fig. 5.4 Contrast-enhanced IR GE sequence 15 min after administration of 0.2 mmol gadolinium-DTPA/kg. Four-chamber view shows marked enhancement of the pericardium (arrows).

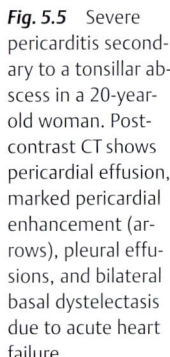

Fig. 5.5 Severe pericarditis secondary to a tonsillar abscess in a 20-year-old woman. Post-contrast CT shows pericardial effusion, marked pericardial enhancement (arrows), pleural effusions, and bilateral basal dystelectasis due to acute heart failure.

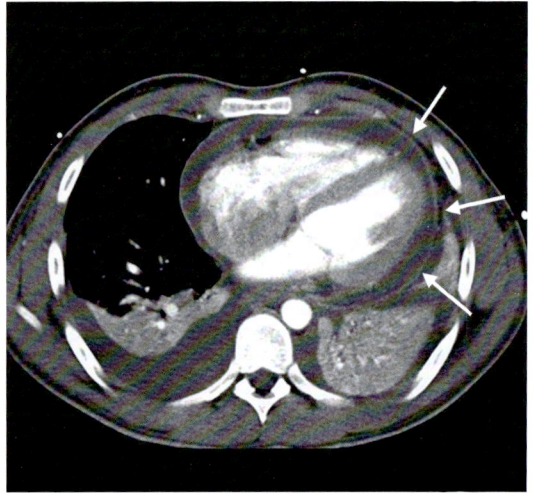

▶ **Course and prognosis**
Usually has a good prognosis • Recurrent pericarditis in 10–15% of cases • Pericardial tamponade with acute heart failure is a rare but life-threatening complication.

▶ **What does the clinician want to know?**
Pericardial effusion and thickening • Inflammatory pericardial changes (MRI) • Impairment of cardiac function.

Differential Diagnosis

Cardiac causes	– Acute coronary syndrome
	– Myocardial infarction
	– Myocarditis
Extracardiac causes	– Aortic dissection
	– Pulmonary embolism
	– Thoracic trauma
Chronic stage	– Constrictive pericarditis
	– RCM

Tips and Pitfalls

Consider pericarditis in the DD of acute chest pain in patients who have a possibly corresponding history. The diagnosis should be established early by the clinical and laboratory findings and ECG. The initial workup should include echocardiography (pericardial effusion).

Selected References

Oyama N et al. Computed tomography and magnetic resonance imaging of the pericardium: anatomy and pathology. Magn Reson Med Sci. 2004; 3: 145–152

Taylor AM, Dymarkowski S, Verbeken EK, Bogaert J. Detection of pericardial inflammation with late-enhancement cardiac magnetic resonance imaging: initial results. Eur Radiol. 2006; 16: 569–574

Definition

▶ **Etiology**
Idiopathic (33%) • Postpericarditic or infectious (19%) • Mechanical (18%, trauma, heart surgery) • Postirradiation (13%, e.g. in Hodgkin disease, breast cancer) • Metabolic (e.g. uremia) • Rheumatic diseases.

▶ **Etiology, pathophysiology, pathogenesis**
Abnormal thickening of the pericardium (normal < 2.5 mm) with fibrosis, calcifications (most pronounced after tuberculosis), and adhesions of the parietal and visceral layers • Impaired diastolic filling of all cardiac chambers with clinical manifestations of right-sided heart failure.

Imaging Signs

▶ **Modality of choice**
MRI • CT may be appropriate for purely morphologic information.

▶ **Chest radiograph and CT findings**
Pericardial calcification or thickening of 3 mm or more (CT) • Pleural effusion • Possible pleural calcification (tuberculosis!).

▶ **Echocardiographic findings**
Pericardial thickening (TEE) • Adhesions • Diastolic dysfunction including paradoxical septal motion • Lateral portions of the pericardium may be difficult to evaluate • Doppler findings often suggest the correct diagnosis.

▶ **MRI findings**
Same as Echocardiographic findings • Better visualization of the pericardium • Also defines the mediastinum • Highest sensitivity of all modalities.

Clinical Aspects

▶ **Typical presentation**
Right-sided heart failure • Dyspnea • Edema • Pleural effusion • Ascites • Hepatosplenomegaly.

▶ **Treatment options**
Treatment of choice is extensive pericardectomy.

▶ **Course and prognosis**
Good prognosis following surgical treatment • Prognosis with conservative treatment is guarded due to progressive right-sided heart failure.

▶ **What does the clinician want to know?**
Pericardial changes • Cardiac functional parameters • Impairment of diastolic function • Signs of right-sided heart failure (including congestion of the venae cavae, hepatic veins and hepatomegaly).

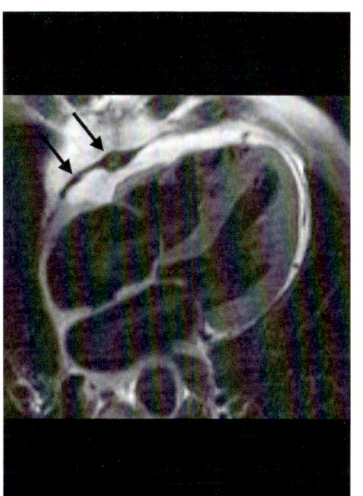

Fig. 5.6 Constrictive pericarditis. T2-weighted dark-blood TSE sequence in the four-chamber plane shows nodular foci of pericardial thickening up to 7 mm in size (arrows).

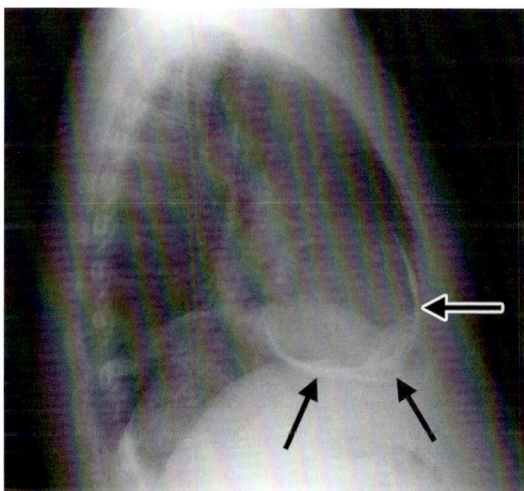

Fig. 5.7 Constrictive pericarditis. Lateral chest radiograph shows flocculent pericardial calcifications (arrows) projected over the cardiac silhouette.

Differential Diagnosis

Other causes of right-sided heart failure	– Pulmonary hypertension with cor pulmonale – Decompensated left-sided heart failure – Liver diseases
Cardiomyopathies	– Important DD: RCM – HCM – Secondary cardiomyopathies with myocardial restriction

Tips and Pitfalls

Constrictive pericarditis without pericardial thickening is present in up to 20% of cases (autopsy statistics). Thus, the absence of a morphologic correlate should always be interpreted within the context of the clinical presentation and functional changes.

Selected References

Hancock EW. Differential diagnosis of restrictive cardiomyopathy and constrictive pericarditis. Heart 2001; 86: 343–349

Ling et al. Constrictive pericarditis in the modern era. Circulation 1999; 100: 1380–1386

Definition

▶ **Epidemiology**
Infectious inflammatory disease of the endocardium • Usually affects the cardiac valves and less commonly the ventricles • Incidence of approximately 5–10/100 000 per year, with regional variations • Acquired and congenital heart disease (aortic or mitral valve disease, VSD) are predisposing • Males are more commonly affected than females.

▶ **Etiology, pathophysiology, pathogenesis**
Involvement of previously damaged cardiac valves in a setting of bacteremia • Eventual destruction of the affected valve • Acute functional impairment • Septic dissemination of causative organisms (mainly streptococci and staphylococci) • Left cardiac valves most commonly affected.

Imaging Signs

▶ **Modality of choice**
Echocardiography.

▶ **Chest radiograph and CT findings**
Pulmonary infiltrates • Mediastinal lymphadenopathy • Whole-body CT shows disseminated septic foci in other organs (liver, spleen, kidneys, brain).

▶ **Echocardiographic findings**
Valvular vegetations (> 90 % sensitivity in TEE) • Quantification of valvular dysfunction (mainly regurgitation) • Assessment of ventricular function.

▶ **MRI findings**
Used rarely for the investigation of an abscess or involvement of other cardiac structures.

▶ **Invasive diagnostic procedures**
Preoperative coronary angiography is indicated in patients aged 40 years or older and in patients with suspected CHD.

Clinical Aspects

▶ **Typical presentation**
– *Acute course:* Septic state (fevers, chills) • Rapid development of heart failure due to valvular dysfunction.
– *Subacute course:* Weight loss • Lethargy • Subfebrile temperatures • Night sweats • Recurrent bacteremia (spiking fever) • Cutaneous septic emboli.

▶ **Treatment options**
Antibiotic therapy • Cardiac valve replacement (may be an emergency indication!) • Surgical abscess drainage • Endocarditis prophylaxis • Anticoagulation.

▶ **Course and prognosis**
Highly variable course ranging from fulminating forms with a rapidly fatal outcome (up to 45 % mortality at 60 days) to subcutaneous disease that runs an undulating course over a period of months.

Fig. 5.8   Acute aortic insufficiency due to endocarditis in a 21-year-old woman. Cine-SSFP image of the LVOT in diastole shows marked regurgitation (small arrows) across the thickened aortic valve (large arrow).

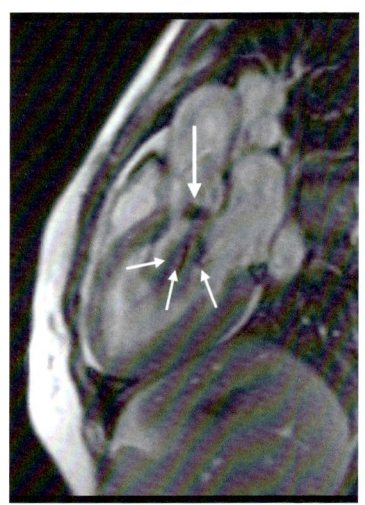

Fig. 5.9   TEE image of a thickened aortic valve (<<<) (after Lambertz H, Lethen H. *Transösophageale Echokardiographie*. Stuttgart: Thieme; 2000).

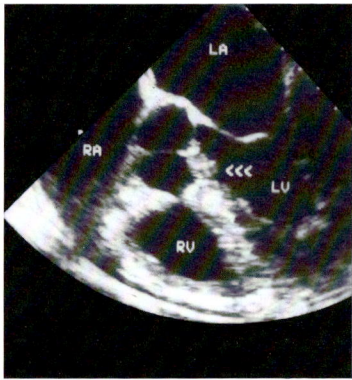

▶ **What does the clinician want to know?**
Valvular vegetations • Valvular dysfunction • Complicating factors (cardiac abscess, septic dissemination).

Differential Diagnosis

Inflammatory heart diseases (myocarditis, pericarditis), rheumatic fever, and collagen diseases.

Tips and Pitfalls

The history is important (infectious focus?). Suspicion of endocarditis warrants immediate hospitalization and prompt diagnostic evaluation.

Selected References

Baddour et al. Infective endocarditis: diagnosis and management. Circulation 2005; 111: e394–433
Lindner JR et al. Diagnostic value of echocardiography in suspected endocarditis: an evaluation based on the pretest probability of disease. Circulation 1996; 93: 730–736

Definition

▶ **Epidemiology**
Eosinophilia of unknown cause (e.g., parasites, drugs, allergies) • Cardiac involvement in approximately 75% of cases • Most common in moderate climatic zones • Predominantly affecting men 20–50 years of age.

▶ **Etiology, pathophysiology, pathogenesis**
Begins as an eosinophilic inflammatory response of the endocardium and subendocardial myocardium, with imaging evidence of thrombi • Later progresses to fibrosis with restriction (endomyocardial fibrosis).

Imaging Signs

▶ **Modality of choice**
Echocardiography.

▶ **Chest radiograph and CT findings**
More manifestations of hypereosinophilic syndrome (e.g., pulmonary infiltrates, mediastinal lymphadenopathy) • Whole-body CT may show disseminated foci and/or thrombotic emboli.

▶ **Echocardiographic and MRI findings**
Valvular dysfunction • Impaired diastolic function (restriction) • Systolic function is initially intact • Increased subendocardial signal intensity on T2-weighted and gadolinium-enhanced images (IR GE sequence).

▶ **Invasive diagnostic procedures**
Myocardial biopsy shows eosinophilic infiltrates • *Caution:* Risk of thrombus dissemination.

Clinical Aspects

▶ **Typical presentation**
General malaise • Lethargy • Fever • Myalgia • Heart failure • Valvular dysfunction • Frequent peripheral emboli (skin, brain, kidneys).

▶ **Treatment options**
Corticosteroids • Tyrosine kinase inhibitors, cytostatics, and interferon • Symptomatic treatment of heart failure • Anticoagulation.

▶ **Course and prognosis**
Good prognosis with early diagnosis and treatment • Heart failure is a limiting factor • Cardiac valve replacement and endomyocardial resection will improve the prognosis.

▶ **What does the clinician want to know?**
Myocardial and valvular function • Signs of restriction • Inflammatory signs (MRI).

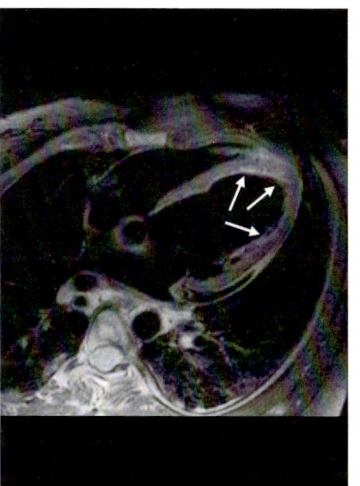

Fig. 5.10   MRI in a 31-year-old woman with recurrent cerebral microemboli. T2-weighted dark-blood TSE sequence in the four-chamber plane shows subendo-cardial foci of increased signal intensity (arrows) corresponding to the postcontrast image.

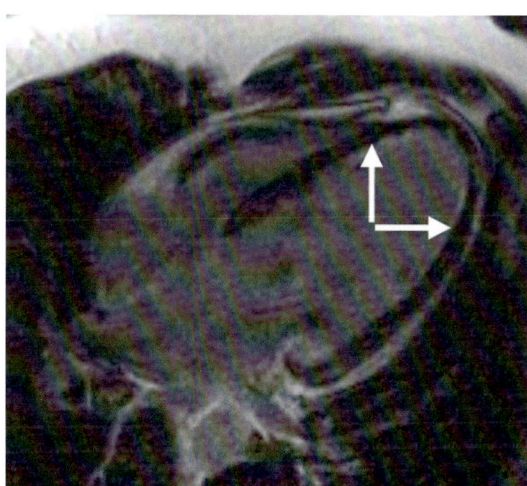

Fig. 5.11   Same patient as in Fig. 5.**10**. Contrast-enhanced IR GE sequence 15 min after administration of 0.2 mmol gadolinium-DTPA/kg in the four-chamber view demonstrates focal enhancement of the endocardium and subendocardial myocardium (arrows).

Differential Diagnosis

Early stage	– Myocarditis
	– Infectious endocarditis
Later stage	– RCM
	– Endomyocardial fibrosis

Tips and Pitfalls

Hypereosinophilic syndrome should be included in the differential diagnosis of unexplained thromboembolism.

Selected References

Plastiras SC et al. Magnetic resonance imaging of the heart in a patient with hypereosinophilic syndrome. Am J Med 2006; 119: 130–132

Weller PF, Bubley GJ: The idiopathic hypereosinophilic syndrome. Blood 1994; 83: 2759–2779

Definition

▶ **Epidemiology**
Postinfarction pericarditis: May occur up to 6 weeks after a myocardial infarction • 50% of cases occur after a transmural myocardial infarction.
Dressler syndrome (postmyocardial infarction syndrome): Occurs weeks to months after a myocardial infarction • The infarction need not be transmural • Develops in less than 5% of myocardial infarctions.

▶ **Etiology, pathophysiology, pathogenesis**
Postinfarction pericarditis: Regional fibrinous inflammation in the infarcted area
Dressler syndrome: Probably has an autoimmune etiology.
A serous or fibrinous hemorrhagic pericardial effusion may develop in both forms.

Imaging Signs

▶ **Modality of choice**
Echocardiography.

▶ **Chest radiograph and CT findings**
Often normal findings • May show signs of pericardial effusion.

▶ **Echocardiographic findings**
May demonstrate pericardial effusion • Myocardial dysfunction in the infarcted area • Dressler syndrome may feature a generalized impairment of diastolic function due to pericardial restriction.

▶ **MRI findings**
Same as Echocardiographic findings • Better visualization of the pericardium.

▶ **Invasive diagnostic procedures**
Coronary angiography should be done to evaluate postinfarction coronary status.

Clinical Aspects

▶ **Typical presentation**
Postinfarction pericarditis: Often does not produce clinical manifestations or is masked by the symptoms of the infarction.
Dressler syndrome: Acute pericarditis with fever • ECG changes • Chest pain • Pericardial rub • Pericardial effusion.

▶ **Treatment options**
Nonsteroidal anti-inflammatory drugs • Steroids should be prescribed in chronic cases (Dressler syndrome).

▶ **Course and prognosis**
Postinfarction pericarditis has a good prognosis • Less common owing to early reperfusion measures (thrombolysis, acute PTCA), which lower the rate of transmural infarction • Pericarditis in Dressler syndrome may recur.

▶ **What does the clinician want to know?**
Pericardial effusion • Inflammatory pericardial changes (MRI) • Cardiac function.

Differential Diagnosis

Cardiac causes	– Acute coronary syndrome
	– Myocardial infarction
	– Myocarditis
Extracardiac causes	– Aortic dissection
	– Pulmonary embolism
Chronic stage	– Constrictive pericarditis
	– RCM

Tips and Pitfalls

A history of infarction yields important information • With a long interval between myocardial infarction and symptom onset, Dressler syndrome might be misinterpreted as an acute coronary syndrome.

Selected References

Indik JH et al. Post-Myocardial Infarction Pericarditis. Curr Treat Options Cardiovasc Med 2000; 2: 351–356

Spodick DH. Pericardial Diseases. In: Braunwald, Zipes, Libby; Heart Disease: A Textbook of Cardiovascular Medicine. Philadelphia: Saunders; 2001

Definition

▶ **Definition**
Arterial hypertension refers to blood pressure elevation above 140/90 mmHg.

▶ **Epidemiology, etiology**
Prevalence: Approximately 20% of adults • Over 90% of patients have primary (essential) hypertension • 5–10% have secondary arterial hypertension (renal, renovascular, endocrine, coarctation of the aorta).

▶ **Pathoanatomy**
Postductal coarctation of the aorta (< 0.1% of all hypertensive patients) is the only cardiovascular cause of arterial hypertension • CHD • Left ventricular hypertrophy • Heart failure (hypertensive cardiomyopathy).

Imaging Signs

▶ **Modality of choice**
Echocardiography.

▶ **Chest radiograph findings**
Often normal • Narrow cardiac silhouette • Rounded left cardiac border • Prominent aortic knob • Aortic elongation and sclerosis • Cardiac decompensation leads to LV enlargement.

▶ **Echocardiographic findings**
Left ventricular hypertrophy (septum > 12 mm) • Aortic ectasia • Diastolic dysfunction • Advanced cases show cardiomegaly and impaired systolic function • TEE may be rewarding in patients with suspected coarctation of the aorta.

▶ **CT findings**
Used as a primary study only in patients with suspected coarctation of the aorta • Demonstrates the vascular complications of arterial hypertension (aortic aneurysm, dissecting aneurysm).

▶ **MRI**
Same as echocardiographic and CT findings • Can be used for accurate assessment and follow-up of myocardial mass.

▶ **Invasive diagnostic procedures**
Coronary angiography can detect coronary stenosis in patients with suspected CHD.

Clinical Aspects

▶ **Typical presentation**
Often asymptomatic • Headache • Vertigo • Angina pectoris • Dyspnea • Epistaxis • Patients with secondary hypertension have symptoms of the underlying disease.

Fig. 6.1 Arterial hypertension in a 63-year-old woman. P-A chest radiograph shows a narrow cardiac silhouette with an elevated apex (arrows) due to myocardial hypertrophy.

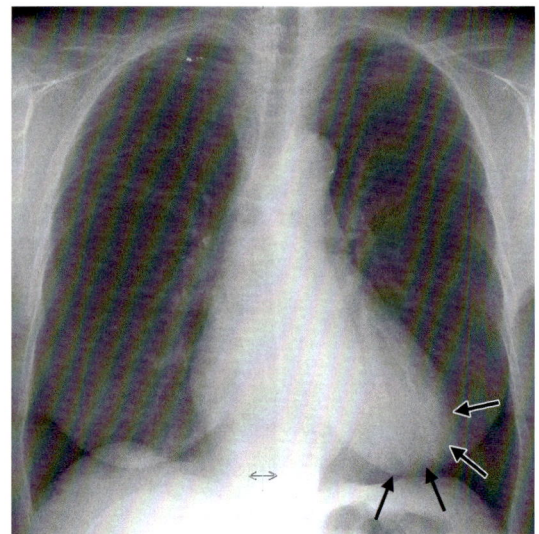

Fig. 6.2 MR image in the same patient as in Fig. 6.**1**. SSFP image in the four-chamber view shows marked, predominantly septal hypertrophy of the LV myocardium.

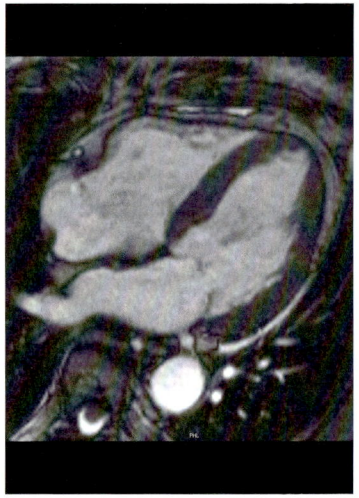

▶ **Treatment options**

Reduction of risk factors in patients with primary hypertension (weight reduction, physical exercise, less alcohol) • Graded drug treatment protocol • Secondary hypertension also requires treatment for the underlying disease (e.g., renal arterial stenosis, pheochromocytoma).

▶ **Course and prognosis**

Prognosis depends on the severity of hypertension and associated risk factors such as atherosclerosis, CHD, cerebral ischemic attacks, aortic aneurysm, and aortic dissection.

▶ **What does the clinician want to know?**

Morphologic and functional evaluation of the heart • Vascular complications • Exclusion of coarctation of the aorta.

Differential Diagnosis

HCM, secondary cardiomyopathies (e.g., amyloidosis, uremic cardiomyopathy), aortic valve stenosis.

Tips and Pitfalls

Secondary hypertension should be excluded before treatment is started.

Selected References

Chobanian AV et al. The Seventh Report of the Joint National Committee on Prevention, Detection, Evaluation, and Treatment of High Blood Pressure. JAMA 2003; 289: 2560–2572

Definition

▶ **Definition**

Increase in pulmonary vascular resistance ● This causes a progressive rise in the mean pulmonary arterial pressure to more than 25 mmHg at rest ● Culminates in right-sided heart failure and premature death.

Classification:

– (*Primary*) idiopathic or familial pulmonary hypertension: Progressive obliteration of small and medium-sized pulmonary arteries.

– (*Secondary*) pulmonary hypertension caused by risk factors or other underlying diseases (various cardiac and pulmonary diseases).

– *Cor pulmonale:* Dilatation and functional impairment of the right ventricle as a result of lung disease with pulmonary hypertension.

▶ **Epidemiology, etiology**

Primary pulmonary hypertension is very rare. Secondary pulmonary hypertension is much more common ● *Possible causes:* Idiopathic ● Collagen diseases ● Portal hypertension ● Medications ● Heart failure ● Valvular heart disease ● COPD ● Interstitial lung disease ● Sleep apnea syndrome ● Pulmonary embolism ● Inflammatory lung diseases.

▶ **Pathoanatomy**

Frequent dilatation of central pulmonary arteries ● Narrowed caliber of small pulmonary arteries (pruning) ● Dilatation and/or hypertrophy of the right ventricle.

Imaging Signs

▶ **Modality of choice**

Echocardiography (heart) ● CT (lung).

▶ **Chest radiograph findings**

Prominent pulmonary segment ● Enlarged central pulmonary arteries ● Rapid tapering of peripheral pulmonary arteries ● Increased lucency of the lung due to decreased vascular markings ● RV hypertrophy (opacification of the retrosternal space in the lateral projection).

▶ **Echocardiographic findings**

Exclusion of left-sided heart failure or valvular heart disease as the cause ● Hypertrophy or dilatation of the right ventricle ● Paradoxical septal motion ● Tricuspid insufficiency ● Estimation of pulmonary arterial pressure based on systolic flow acceleration at the tricuspid valve.

▶ **CT findings**

Evidence of lung disease (e.g., COPD, emphysema, interstitial lung disease) or pulmonary embolism ● Dimensions of the right ventricle and pulmonary vessels.

▶ **MRI findings**

Good morphologic and functional evaluation of the right ventricle and pulmonary vessels in patients with suspected cor pulmonale ● Time-resolved contrast-

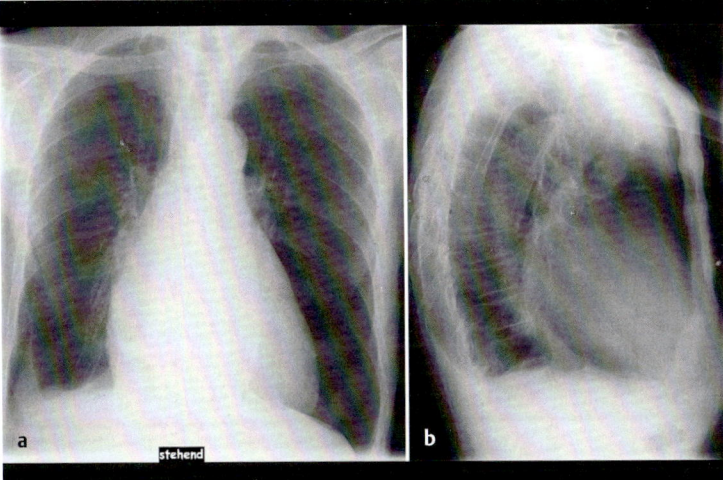

Fig. 6.3 a, b   P-A (**a**) and lateral chest radiograph (**b**) in a 73-year-old man with pulmonary emphysema and pulmonary hypertension demonstrate pruning of the hilar vessels, RV dilatation, and right pleural effusion. The RV is broadly apposed to the sternum in the lateral projection.

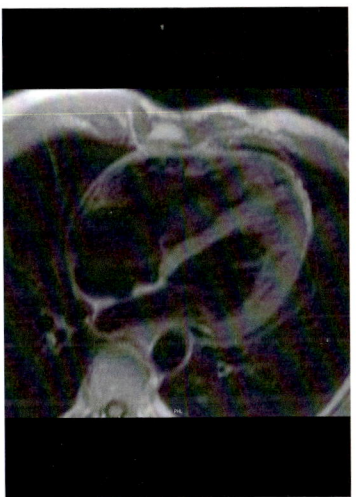

Fig. 6.4   MR image of pulmonary hypertension in a 44-year-old man. Dark-blood T1-weighted TSE sequence in the four-chamber view shows marked dilatation of the RA and RV with a normal appearance of the left heart.

enhanced MRA can evaluate the great vessels and lung perfusion in patients with suspected pulmonary embolism.

▶ **Ventilation–perfusion nuclear medicine**
Used only to investigate presumptive pulmonary embolism • May show a discrepancy between perfused and ventilated segments.

▶ **Invasive diagnostic procedures**
Pulmonary angiography and right-heart catheterization are indicated only in patients selected for thromboendarterectomy or to quantify pulmonary hypertension at rest and during exercise • Detection of sustained pulmonary hypertension with increased resistance in the small arteries and arterioles (diastolic pulmonary arterial pressure is higher than pulmonary capillary wedge pressure).

Clinical Aspects

▶ **Typical presentation**
Level of symptomatology is often mild • Dyspnea • Weakness • Syncope • Vertigo • Sinus tachycardia • Cyanosis.

▶ **Treatment options**
Conservative: Oxygen administration • Treatment of infection • Treatment of underlying disease • Oral anticoagulants • Diuretics • Vasodilators (e.g., calcium antagonists, sildenafil, bosentan, prostaglandin analogs).
Surgical: Chronic pulmonary emboli can be surgically managed by thromboendarterectomy or lung transplantation.

▶ **Course and prognosis**
Primary pulmonary hypertension has a 3-year survival rate less than 50% • Prognosis of secondary pulmonary hypertension depends on the underlying disease and degree of severity.

▶ **What does the clinician want to know?**
Degree of right-heart overload (RV hypertrophy or dilatation, diameter of vena cava and hepatic veins, cardiac cirrhosis) • RV function • Pulmonary insufficiency • Etiologic signs (pulmonary status).

Tips and Pitfalls

Pulmonary angiography can lead to acute right-heart decompensation in patients with severe pulmonary arterial hypertension with a systolic pulmonary arterial pressure above 60 mmHg. Thus, rigorous criteria should be applied in selecting patients for this procedure.

Selected References

Galie N et al. Guidelines on diagnosis and treatment of pulmonary arterial hypertension. The Task Force on Diagnosis and Treatment of Pulmonary Arterial Hypertension of the European Society of Cardiology. Eur Heart J 2004; 25: 2243–2278

Yilmaz E et al. Accuracy and feasibility of dynamic contrast-enhanced 3D MR imaging in the assessment of lung perfusion: comparison with Tc-99 MAA perfusion scintigraphy. Clin Radiol 2005; 60: 905–913

Definition

▶ **Definition, classification**

Condition in which thrombi have dislodged and embolized, causing obstruction of pulmonary arteries.

Grading of severity (ESC 2000):
– Grade 1
  Massive pulmonary embolism with shock and/or hypotension.
– Grade 2
  Nonmassive pulmonary embolism.
– Grade 2a
  Submassive pulmonary embolism, i.e., nonmassive pulmonary embolism with signs of right-heart overload.

▶ **Epidemiology, etiology**

Incidence of approximately 0.5 cases/1000/year ● Pulmonary emboli are common in hospitalized patients (approximately 1–2%) but often go undetected ● More than 90% of thrombi originate in regions drained by the inferior vena cava ● Predisposing factors are immobility, fractures, surgical operations, malignancies, heart failure, and coagulation disorders.

▶ **Pathoanatomy**

Hemodynamically significant obstruction of the pulmonary arteries imposes an acute overload on the right heart.

Imaging Signs

▶ **Modality of choice**

CT.

▶ **Chest radiograph findings**

A normal chest radiograph does not exclude pulmonary embolism ● Atelectasis (< 70%) ● Small pleural effusions (< 50%) ● Wedge-shaped subpleural density (< 35%) ● Elevation of the hemidiaphragm (< 25%) ● Focal pulmonary oligemia distal to the embolism (Westermark sign, 10%), dilatation of the RV and pulmonary artery (< 10%).

▶ **Echocardiographic findings**

With a hemodynamically significant pulmonary embolism, more than 30% of the pulmonary circulation is occluded ● Dilatation and hypokinesia of the RV ● Paradoxical septal motion ● Tricuspid insufficiency ● Increased pulmonary arterial pressure ● Dilatation of the inferior vena cava ● Rarely, echo may detect thrombi in the RA or RV.

▶ **CT findings**

Can define thromboembolic masses in the pulmonary circulation ● RV enlargement due to a hemodynamically significant pulmonary embolism ● Small peripheral emboli may escape detection, but most have little clinical significance.
Qanadli obstruction index: $\Sigma\,(n \times d)/40 \times 100$, where n = segments (1–20), d = degree of obstruction (0 = clear, 1 = partial occlusion, 2 = total occlusion).

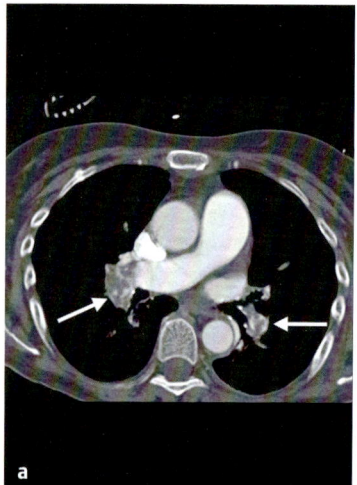

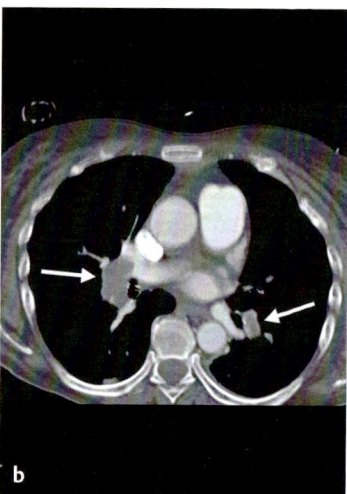

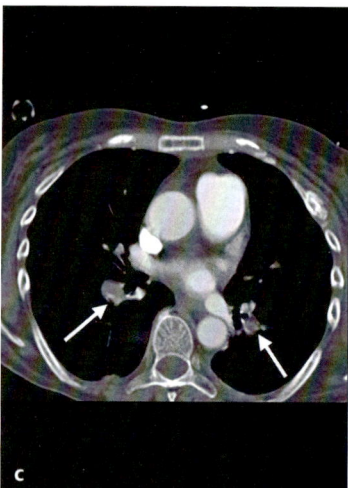

Fig. 6.5 a–c Acute pulmonary embolism. Contrast-enhanced CT scan demonstrates thrombi in both central pulmonary arteries (arrows).

▶ **MRI findings**
Same as CT and echocardiographic findings ● Too time-consuming in acute situations ● Otherwise, an equally good alternative.

▶ **Nuclear medicine**
Perfusion scanning reveals perfusion defects caused by significant embolism ● A normal scan excludes pulmonary embolism with reasonable confidence.

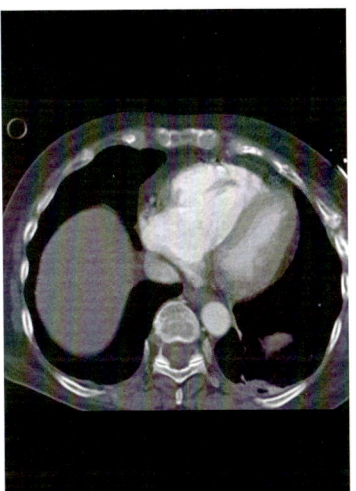

Fig. 6.6 Acute pulmonary embolism. Contrast-enhanced CT scan shows marked right-heart overload with displacement of the interventricular septum toward the left side due to the increased right ventricular pressure.

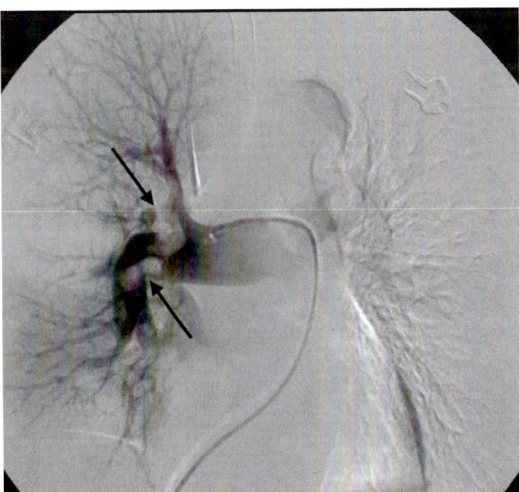

Fig. 6.7 Selective DSA of the right pulmonary artery prior to mechanical fragmentation. Partially occlusive thrombi are seen at the bifurcation of the main trunk (arrows).

▶ **Invasive diagnostic procedures**

CT has replaced angiography as the "gold standard" ● Interventional (mechanical) fragmentation of the embolic mass may be followed by (selective) lytic therapy ● The interventional procedure may be preceded by angiography.

Clinical Aspects

▶ **Typical presentation**
Dyspnea (85%) • Chest pain varying with respiratory excursions (85%) • Sinus tachycardia (60%) • Anxiety • Chest tightness (60%) • Cough (50%) • Vertigo • Syncope • Shock (15%).

▶ **Treatment options**
- *Symptomatic:* Oxygen administration • Inotropic agents • Vasopressors • Ventilation if required.
- *Anticoagulation:* Heparin • Fibrinolytics • Long-term oral anticoagulation.
- *Invasive:* Fragmentation of the thrombus • Surgical embolectomy • Vena cava filter to prevent recurrence (adapted selection criteria).

▶ **Course and prognosis**
Prognosis depends on severity • 90-day mortality is 54% for massive pulmonary embolism and 15% for nonmassive pulmonary embolism.

▶ **What does the clinician want to know?**
Establish the diagnosis • Exclude other diagnoses • Embolism grade and degree of right-heart overload • Location of thrombosis.

Differential Diagnosis

Other causes of dyspnea	– Pulmonary edema
	– Asthma attack, COPD
	– Pneumothorax
	– Pneumonia
	– Psychogenic hyperventilation
Other causes of chest pain	– Acute coronary syndrome
	– Aortic dissection
	– Pleurisy
	– Pericarditis
	– Vertebrogenic pain
	– Esophagitis

Tips and Pitfalls

The decision regarding lytic therapy is based on clinical parameters and the load on the right heart. This decision is not based directly on the extent of the thrombi (e.g., as determined by CT).

Selected References

Qanadli SD et al. New CT index to quantify arterial obstruction in pulmonary embolism: comparison with angiographic index and echocardiography. AJR Am J Roentgenol 2001; 176: 1415–1420

Torbicki A et al.: Diagnosis and management of pulmonary embolism. European Heart Journal 2000, 21: 1301–1336

Definition

▶ **Epidemiology**
Most common intracardiac mass • Variable etiology.

▶ **Etiology, pathophysiology, pathogenesis**
The etiology varies according to the location of the thrombus:
   – LA: Atrial fibrillation • Mitral stenosis.
   – LV: In 40–60% of patients with anterior myocardial infarction without anti-coagulation.
   – RA: Poor cardiac function • Atrial fibrillation • Central venous catheter or pacemaker lead • Transvenous ablation • Rheumatic tricuspid stenosis • Cardiac surgery • Cardiomyopathy • Tumor thrombus extension from renal-cell or hepatocellular carcinoma through the inferior vena cava.
   – RV: Rare • Etiology same as RA thrombus.

Imaging Signs

▶ **Modality of choice**
Echocardiography.

▶ **Chest radiograph findings**
Often normal • May show calcification of the thrombus or of a postinfarction scar • LV enlargement due to a ventricular aneurysm.

▶ **Echocardiographic findings**
Iso- to hyperechoic floating, pedunculated, or mural mass • Often found in a hypokinetic area (anterior or apical).

▶ **CT findings**
Hypodense mass with smooth or irregular margins that does not enhance after contrast administration • Mural or pedunculated • Floating thrombi may not be detected • ECG-triggered multidetector CT can detect thrombi in the left heart with high sensitivity • The right heart is often more difficult to evaluate.

▶ **MRI findings**
Same as echocardiographic and CT findings • Iso- to hyperintense on T1-weighted and T2-weighted images, depending on the age of the thrombus • Absence of contrast enhancement (!) may provide the only differentiating criterion from other tumors.

▶ **Invasive diagnostic procedures**
Ventriculogram shows a filling defect that may be free-floating • Usually detected incidentally during coronary angiography.

Clinical Aspects

▶ **Typical presentation**
   – *Left heart:* Stroke • Peripheral emboli.
   – *Right heart:* Pulmonary embolism.

▶ **Treatment options**
Treatment of underlying disease (mitral stenosis, CHD) • Anticoagulation.

Fig. 7.1 Patient following an anterior wall infarction with an anterior wall aneurysm. SSFP sequence, long-axis view parallel to the septum shows an apical wall adherent thrombus of the left ventricle in the area of the aneurysm (arrows).

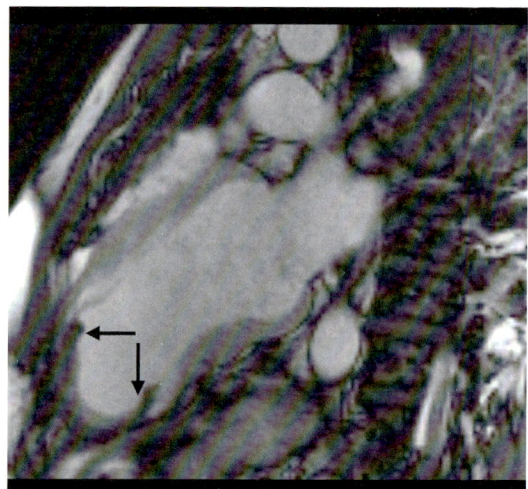

Fig. 7.2 Same patient as in Fig. 7.1. SSFP image, four-chamber view.

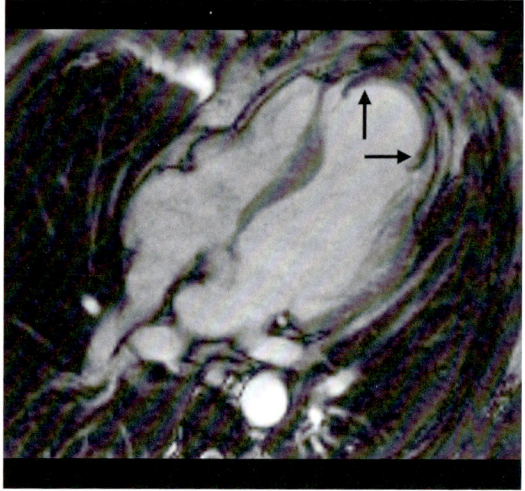

▶ **Course and prognosis**
Mural thrombus formation 48–72 hours after a myocardial infarction suggests poor prognosis due to associated complications.

▶ **What does the clinician want to know?**
Location and size of the thrombotic material • Attachment to the vessel wall • Etiology.

Differential Diagnosis

Benign tumor	– Myxoma (most common cardiac tumor): usually shows different signal and enhancement characteristics on MRI
Malignant tumor *(metastasis, sarcoma)*	– Infiltration of the myocardium
	– Pericardial invasion
	– Metastasis

Tips and Pitfalls

Thrombi are often detected incidentally and are occasionally missed in sectional imaging studies.

Selected References

Koca V et al. Left atrial thrombus detection with multiplane transesophageal echocardiography: an echocardiographic study with surgical verification. J Heart Valve Dis 1999; 8: 63–66

Tatli S, Lipton MJ. CT for intracardiac thrombi and tumors. Int J Cardiovasc Imaging 2005; 21: 115–131

Definition

▶ **Epidemiology**
Most common primary cardiac tumor (approximately 50%) • 90% of patients are between 30 and 60 years of age • Occurs sporadically, but patients with Carney complex are predisposed • More common in females than in males (4:1).

▶ **Etiology, pathophysiology, pathogenesis**
Originates from embryonic cells • Common in the left atrium (60–80%) • Less common in the right atrium (20–25%) • Usually arises from the interatrial septum • May also be situated on cardiac valves or the eustachian valve (at termination of inferior vena cava).

Imaging Signs

▶ **Modality of choice**
Echocardiography.

▶ **Chest radiograph findings**
Usually normal • May show dilatation of the affected atrium • Tumor mass and/or tumor calcification.

▶ **Echocardiographic findings**
Lobulated or villous, sessile or pedunculated mass of high echogenicity • Frequent thrombotic deposits • Tumor prolapses through the tricuspid or mitral valve during cardiac contractions, with associated regurgitation or obstruction.

▶ **CT findings**
Heterogeneous appearance • Most commonly appears as a hypodense mass with cystic, necrotic, or hemorrhagic inclusions • Calcification may be seen (16%).

▶ **MRI findings**
Same as echocardiographic and CT findings • Hypo- to isointense on T1-weighted images • Usually hyperintense on T2-weighted images • Heterogeneous enhancement pattern is an important differentiating criterion from thrombi.

Clinical Aspects

▶ **Typical presentation**
Asymptomatic in 20% of cases • Symptoms similar to endocarditis (fatigue, arthralgia, weight loss, anemia, fever) • Frequent CNS symptoms or peripheral emboli (40%, caused by dislodged thrombi) • Cardiac arrhythmias (20%) • Impaired cardiac function is marked by dyspnea, peripheral edema, hepatic congestion, and ascites.

▶ **Treatment options**
Surgical resection • Valve reconstruction may be indicated.

▶ **Course and prognosis**
Good prognosis • 5% incidence of postoperative recurrence, possibly with a multifocal distribution (cardiac, cerebral).

▶ **What does the clinician want to know?**
Size • Location • Impairment of valve function • Obstruction • Thrombi.

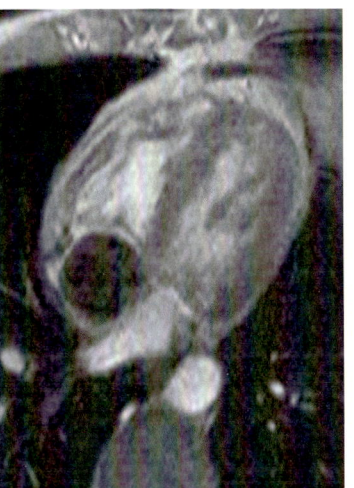

Fig. 7.3 T1-weighted GRE sequence of atrial myxoma. Four-chamber view shows a well-circumscribed hypointense mass in the right atrium abutting the interatrial septum. Histological examination confirmed myxoma.

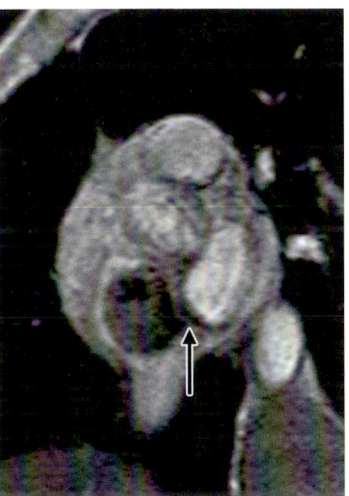

Fig. 7.4 Same patient as in Fig. 7.**3**. T1-weighted GRE sequence, short-axis view through the atrium shows that the myxoma is in contact with the interatrial septum (arrow).

Differential Diagnosis

Most important DD: thrombus	– Often associated with atrial fibrillation and mitral stenosis
	– Often located on the posterior or lateral wall of the LA
	– DD should be narrowed by contrast-enhanced MRI in doubtful cases
Carney complex	– Autosomal dominant
	– Multiple myxomas (cardiac, cutaneous, mammary)
	– Skin pigmentation
	– Cushing syndrome and other manifestations including Sertoli cell tumor
Other (malignant) tumors	– Broad area of attachment
	– Different signal characteristics (MRI)

Tips and Pitfalls

Differentiation from metastases and thrombi can be difficult • Diagnosis is aided in these cases by MRI • Some cases cannot be diagnosed before surgical resection.

Selected References

Grebenc ML et al. Primary cardiac and pericardial neoplasms: Radiologic-pathologic correlation. Radiographics 2000; 20(4): 1073–1103

Ipek G et al. Surgical management of cardiac myxoma. J Card Surg 2005; 20: 300–304

Definition

▶ **Epidemiology**
Approximately 60 cases have been described worldwide • No age predilection • Detected incidentally on the basis of cardiac murmurs or abnormalities on chest radiograph • Much less common than lipomatous hypertrophy of the interatrial septum.

▶ **Etiology, pathophysiology, pathogenesis**
Differentiated fat cells • Large tumor mass (up to 4.8 kg has been reported) • Often arises from the epicardium • Extension into the pericardial sac.

Imaging Signs

▶ **Modality of choice**
Echocardiography, MRI.

▶ **Chest radiograph findings**
Often normal • May form a radiographically visible mass • Large tumors cause enlargement of the cardiac silhouette • Hemodynamically significant lesions may produce signs of heart failure.

▶ **Echocardiographic findings**
Hyperechoic intracardiac or pericardial mass • Mobile or sessile • Intraluminal determination of cardiac and valvular function.

▶ **CT findings**
Homogeneous, encapsulated tumor that is isodense to fat • No calcifications • Hemorrhagic or necrotic areas.

▶ **MRI findings**
High T1-weighted signal intensity (same as fat) • Nonenhancing • Suppressed signal intensity on fat-suppressed sequences is pathognomonic for lipoma.

▶ **Invasive diagnostic procedures**
Invasive tests do not add diagnostic information.

Clinical Aspects

▶ **Typical presentation**
Frequently asymptomatic with no impairment of cardiac function • May present with nonspecific symptoms • Dyspnea • Arrhythmias (atrial fibrillation, ventricular tachycardia, AV block) • Large lipomas cause impairment of cardiac function.

▶ **Treatment options, course, and prognosis**
Surgical resection • Good postoperative prognosis.

▶ **What does the clinician want to know?**
Location (intracardiac, pericardial) • Differential diagnosis • Impairment of cardiac function • Compression of ventricles or atria.

Fig. 7.5 Interatrial lipoma in a 54-year-old man (incidental finding). Axial contrast-enhanced CT shows a hypodense mass of fat attenuation (arrow).

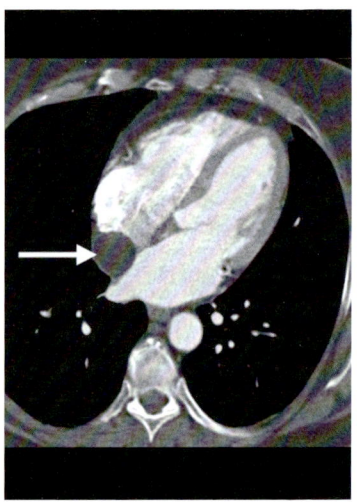

Fig. 7.6 Same patient as in Fig. 7.**5**. Dark-blood T1-weighted TSE sequence in the four-chamber view shows a hyperintense mass of fat attenuation bordering the posterior aspect of the interatrial septum (arrow).

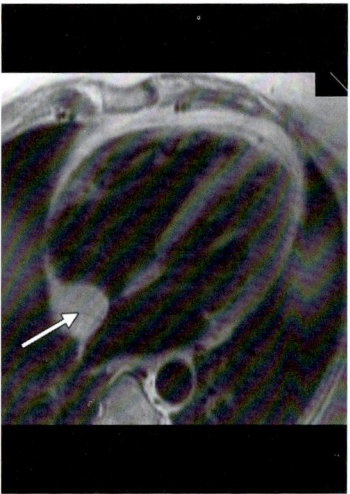

Differential Diagnosis

Rhabdomyosarcoma in children	– Fibroma: Solitary, ventricular, calcified, different contrast characteristics in CT and MRI – Rhabdomyoma: Multiple masses – Tuberous sclerosis
Fatty infiltration of the atrial septum	– Fatty infiltration more than 2 cm in transverse diameter – Common in overweight patients with atrial fibrillation – Spares the fossa ovalis

Tips and Pitfalls

Differentiation is required from cardiac lipomatosis and lipomatous interatrial hypertrophy.

Selected References

Nadra I et al. Lipomatous hypertrophy of the interatrial septum: a commonly misdiagnosed mass often leading to unnecessary cardiac surgery. Heart 2004; 90: e66

Salanitri JC, Pereles FS. Cardiac lipoma and lipomatous hypertrophy of the interatrial septum: cardiac magnetic resonance imaging findings. J Comput Assist Tomogr 2004; 28: 852–856

Definition

▶ **Epidemiology**
Synonyms: Fibromatosis, fibrous hamartoma, fibroelastic hamartoma • Occurs predominantly in children under 10 years of age (40% during first year of life) • Second most common benign primary tumor in this age group, after rhabdomyoma • Patients with Gorlin syndrome are predisposed.

▶ **Etiology, pathophysiology, pathogenesis**
Most fibromas occur in the ventricular myocardium, showing a predilection for the septum and lateral wall of the LV • Up to 5 cm in diameter • May narrow the ventricular lumen.

Imaging Signs

▶ **Modality of choice**
Echocardiography.

▶ **Chest radiograph findings**
Often normal • May show a bulge in the cardiac outline • Cardiomegaly or focal cardiac mass • Calcium deposits • Possible signs of heart failure • Pleural or pericardial effusion.

▶ **Echocardiographic findings**
Isoechoic intramyocardial mass • Often large • Noncontractile • May cause impairment of cardiac function (e.g., by narrowing the outflow tract).

▶ **CT findings**
Intramyocardial mass • Hypo- or isodense to the myocardium • Often calcified • No cystic, necrotic, or hemorrhagic areas • Exclusion of metastases.

▶ **MRI findings**
Isointense to myocardium on T1-weighted images • May exhibit low T2-weighted signal intensity • Same enhancement characteristics as myocardium.

Clinical Aspects

▶ **Typical presentation**
Frequent cardiac arrhythmias • Approximately 30% of patients have no impairment of cardiac function • Incidental finding on the basis of ECG changes, cardiac murmurs, or abnormalities on chest radiograph.

▶ **Treatment options**
Surgical intervention with (partial) resection in symptomatic cases.

▶ **Course and prognosis**
Usually good, depending on tumor size and location.

▶ **What does the clinician want to know?**
Relationship of the tumor to surrounding structures • Impairment of blood flow or cardiac function • Pericardial effusion • Exclusion of metastases.

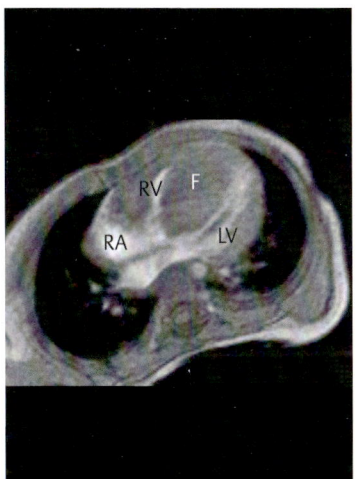

Fig. 7.7 Extensive fibroma in the interventricular septum and RVOT of a 13-month-old girl. ECG-triggered GRE sequence. Four-chamber view at end diastole shows a mass (F) that is isointense to the myocardium and is narrowing the RV lumen.

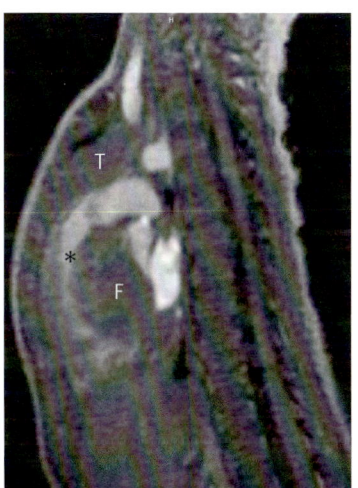

Fig. 7.8 Same patient as in Fig. 7.**7**. ECG-triggered GRE sequence in the plane of the RVOT at end diastole reveals marked narrowing of the outflow tract (*) by the fibroma (F). T, thymus.

Differential Diagnosis

HCM	– May have same imaging features
	– No short-term increase in myocardial thickening
Rhabdomyoma in children	– Fibroma: Solitary, ventricular, calcified
	– Rhabdomyoma: Multiple masses, tuberous sclerosis

Tips and Pitfalls

Children with a new cardiac murmur or abnormal findings on chest radiograph should undergo immediate echocardiography.

Selected References

Kiaffas MG et al. Magnetic resonance imaging evaluation of cardiac tumor characteristics in infants and children. Am J Cardiol 2002; 89: 1229–1233

Kim TH et al. Perinatal sonographic diagnosis of cardiac fibroma with MR imaging correlation. AJR Am J Roentgenol 2002; 178: 727–729

Definition

▶ **Epidemiology**
Second most common benign primary cardiac tumor (approximately 10%) •
Males and females are affected equally • Average age at diagnosis is 60 years •
Occasionally detected incidentally at echo, cardiac surgery, or autopsy.

▶ **Etiology, pathophysiology, pathogenesis**
Etiology is uncertain • 90% of fibroelastomas arise from cardiac valves: aortic
(29%), mitral (25%), pulmonary (13%), and tricuspid (17%).

Imaging Signs

▶ **Modality of choice**
Echocardiography.

▶ **Chest radiograph and CT findings**
Generally the chest radiograph does not add diagnostic information • Mass can
be detected by contrast-enhanced ECG-triggered multidetector CT • CT can exclude metastases in cases with an equivocal DD.

▶ **Echocardiographic findings**
May demonstrate a pedunculated, mobile, hyperechoic tumor • Poorly demar-
cated from surrounding blood • Fibroelastomas have a "sea anemone" appearance and may reach 4 cm in size • Rarely show calcifications • Thrombotic deposits may be found.

▶ **MRI findings**
Tumor has low T1-weighted signal intensity and enhances after gadolinium administration • Because of its location on cardiac valves, the tumor may be defin-
able only on cine sequences with high temporal resolution.

Clinical Aspects

▶ **Typical presentation**
May be asymptomatic, especially when located in the right heart • Tumors in the
left heart may cause embolic complications due to thrombi or tumor fragments •
Chest pain • Dyspnea • Arrhythmias.

▶ **Treatment options**
Surgical resection with valve reconstruction or replacement.

▶ **Course and prognosis**
Good • Tumors do not recur after operative removal.

▶ **What does the clinician want to know?**
Location • Specific diagnosis (myxoma, thrombus, other tumor, evidence of malignancy) • Valvular dysfunction • Cardiac function • Pericardial effusion.

Tumors and Other Masses

Fig. 7.9 Fat-saturated T1-weighted TSE sequence after gadolinium-DTPA administration in a 42-year-old man who experienced an embolic TIA. Image in the plane of the LVOT demonstrates an enhancing mass on the left coronary valve cusp (arrow). Histological examination after valvular replacement confirmed fibroelastoma.

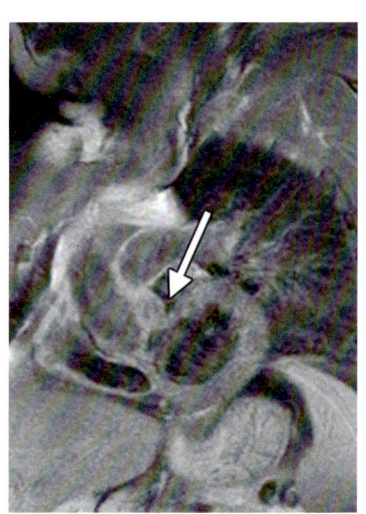

Differential Diagnosis

Thrombus	– Fibroelastoma appears on echocardiography as a pedunculated mass based on a valve – Poorly delineated from surrounding blood
Myxoma	– Often hyperintense on contrast-enhanced T2-weighted images – May be indistinguishable from papillary fibroelastoma
Bacterial vegetation	– Destruction of the affected valve (regurgitation, cardiac murmur) – Fever

Tips and Pitfalls

Echocardiography is always indicated in patients with a history of recurrent and unexplained thromboembolic events • The differential diagnosis of cardiac valve masses should include papillary fibroelastoma.

Selected References

Araoz PA et al. CT and MR Imaging of Benign Primary Cardiac Neoplasms with Echocardiographic Correlation. RadioGraphics 2000; 20: 1303–1319

Bootsveld A et al. Incidental finding of a papillary fibroelastoma on the aortic valve in 16 slice multi-detector row computed tomography. Heart 2004; 90: e35

Sparrow PJ. MR Imaging of Cardiac Tumors. RadioGraphics 2005; 25: 1255–1276

Definition

▶ **Epidemiology**
Congenital malformation ● Evagination of pericardium during early cardiac development ● Rarely symptomatic ● Usually an incidental finding.

▶ **Etiology, pathophysiology, pathogenesis**
Most commonly located in the right cardiophrenic angle ● Other sites are less common but may be seen ● Most pericardial cysts are not septate.

Imaging Signs

▶ **Modality of choice**
Echocardiography.

▶ **Echocardiographic findings**
Well-circumscribed, echo-free paracardiac mass ● No internal echoes ● Absence of perfusion in Doppler ultrasound ● Usually does not impair cardiac function.

▶ **Chest radiograph findings**
Homogeneous paracardiac mass ● Usually abuts the right posterolateral aspect of the cardiac silhouette with negative silhouette sign.

▶ **MRI and CT findings**
CT: Well-circumscribed mass ● Usually smaller than 3 cm ● Thin wall ● Liquid attenuation values in range of 20–50 HU ● No contrast enhancement ● No septa.
MRI: Hyperintense on T2-weighted images ● Iso- to hyperintense on T1-weighted images (protein-rich fluid) ● No contrast enhancement.

Clinical Aspects

▶ **Typical presentation**
Frequently asymptomatic ● Detected incidentally on the chest radiograph ● Cyst may impinge on neighboring organs, causing chest pain, dyspnea, and cough.

▶ **Treatment options**
Treatment is rarely necessary ● Surgical (thoracoscopic) removal or percutaneous drainage of the cyst contents.

▶ **Course and prognosis**
Benign course ● Complications are rare and may relate to therapeutic measures: Cyst rupture, superinfection, pericardial tamponade.

▶ **What does the clinician want to know?**
Location of the cyst ● Exclusion of other masses.

Fig. 7.10 Pericardial cyst. Axial T1-weighted image shows a pericardial cyst (*) in the right paracardiac region with moderate, homogeneous signal intensity. The cyst has smooth margins and does not contain internal septa.

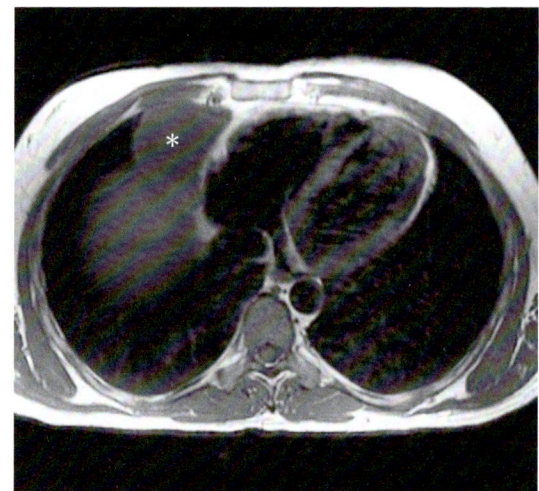

Fig. 7.11 Axial fat-saturated T2-weighted image shows a pericardial cyst of uniformly high signal intensity in the right paracardiac region.

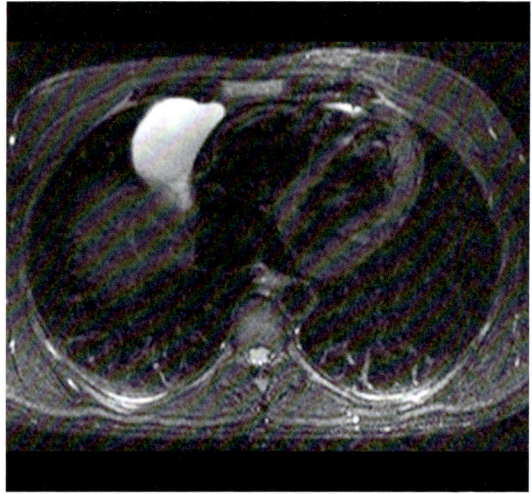

Differential Diagnosis

Malignant mediastinal tumors	– Solid mass
	– Enhances on postcontrast CT and MRI
	– Invasion of adjacent structures
	– Possible metastases (lung, lymph nodes)
Bronchogenic cyst	– Borders on the carina (> 50%), trachea, or esophagus
	– May contain cartilaginous elements

Tips and Pitfalls

Pericardial cyst should be included in the differential diagnosis of patients with a malignant underlying disease and a cystic paracardiac mass.

Selected References

Patel J. Pericardial cyst: case reports and a literature review. Echocardiography 2004; 21: 269–272

Wang ZJ et al. CT and MR imaging of pericardial disease. RadioGraphics 2003; 23: 167–180

Definition

▶ **Epidemiology**

Second most common tumor of the heart and pericardium • Far more common than primary cardiac tumors (prevalence of 1.23% v 0.056% in autopsy series) • Cardiac metastases are found in 10–12% of patients with autopsy-confirmed malignant disease.

Common primary tumors that metastasize to the heart are: Bronchial carcinoma (36%); tumors such as lymphoma, leukemia, and Kaposi sarcoma (20%); breast carcinoma (7%); and esophageal carcinoma (6%).

▶ **Routes of metastasis**

– *Retrograde lymphatic spread:* Common • Small tumor deposits found mainly in the epicardium • Pericardial effusion is common due to obstruction of lymphatic drainage.

– *Hematogenous spread:* Coronary arteries • Tumor deposits found mainly in the myocardium • Frequently associated with pulmonary metastases.

– *Direct infiltration:* By bronchial, esophageal, and breast cancer or mediastinal lymphoma.

– *Transvenous metastasis:* Renal-cell and hepatocellular carcinoma are particularly apt to metastasize through the inferior vena cava.

Imaging Signs

▶ **Modality of choice**

Echocardiography.

▶ **Chest radiograph findings**

Often normal • Cardiomegaly or focal cardiac mass • Possible signs of heart failure • Pleural or pericardial effusion • Other thoracic metastases.

▶ **Echocardiographic findings**

Mass • Precise localization • Evaluation of cardiac function • Assessment of possible ventricular or valvular dysfunction • Pericardial effusion.

▶ **CT findings**

Although less sensitive in detecting a cardiac mass, CT can accurately define its relationship to extracardiac structures and detect additional metastases.

▶ **MRI findings**

No specific differentiating criteria from other tumors • Findings comparable to echocardiography and CT, with high diagnostic accuracy • The other modalities are usually adequate for the initial workup. MRI is used mainly to narrow the DD and monitor treatment response.

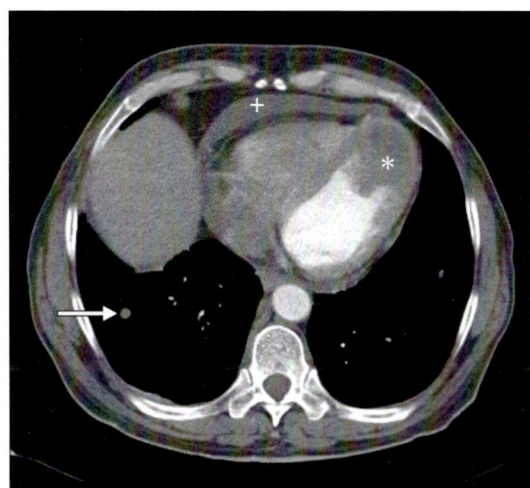

Fig. 7.12 Stage IV metastatic melanoma in a 44-year-old man. Contrast-enhanced axial CT shows a hypodense mass at the LV apex (*, metastasis), a malignant pericardial effusion (+), and a pulmonary metastasis (arrow).

Clinical Aspects

▶ **Typical presentation**

Often asymptomatic initially • Approximately 30% of patients have subsequent impairment of cardiac function (usually due to pericardial effusion) • Cough • Dyspnea (cardiac or due to pericardial effusion) • Chest pain • Peripheral edema • Arrhythmias (infiltration of neurovascular structures) • Heart failure.

▶ **Treatment options**

Pericardial effusion: Pericardial fenestration or sclerotherapy • Radiotherapy • Resection or partial resection is an option in selected patients with impaired cardiac function • Chemotherapy or radiotherapy may be indicated, depending on the primary tumor.

▶ **Course and prognosis**

Death from cardiac metastasis occurs in approximately one-third of cases • Possible causes of death are pericardial tamponade, heart failure, and infiltration of coronary arteries or the sinus node • Poor prognosis with malignant pericardial effusion.

▶ **What does the clinician want to know?**

Detection and localization of metastasis • Impairment of cardiac function • Infiltration of surrounding structures • Pericardial effusion.

Differential Diagnosis

Cardiac thrombi — Tumor and fresh thrombus have high T2-weighted SI on MRI
— Tumor shows contrast enhancement

Pericardial effusion — Pericarditis due to infection, radiation, or chemotherapy
— Pericardiocentesis may be necessary for definitive diagnosis

Tips and Pitfalls

Cardiac metastases are often missed by staging CT! • Watch out for pericardial and cardiac involvement in patients with malignant melanoma, bronchial carcinoma, breast carcinoma, or pleural metastasis • Because metastases are the most common cardiac malignancies, an extracardiac primary tumor should be excluded during the initial workup.

Selected References

Abraham KP et al. Neoplasms metastatic to the heart: review of 3314 consecutive autopsies. Am J Cardiovasc Pathol 1990; 3: 195–198

Chiles C et al. Metastatic Involvement of the Heart and Pericardium: CT and MR Imaging. RadioGraphics 2001; 21: 439–449

MacGee W. Metastatic and invasive tumors involving the heart in a geriatric population: a necropsy study. Virchows Arch A Pathol Anat Histopathol 1991; 419: 183–189

Definition

▶ **Epidemiology**
Most common malignant tumor, comprising approximately 37% of primary cardiac malignancies ● More common in males than in females (2:1) ● Variable occurrence ● Typically affects middle-aged men.

▶ **Etiology, pathophysiology, pathogenesis**
Endothelial tumor ● Most commonly occurs in the free wall of the RA (80%) ● Tumor may infiltrate the pericardium.

Imaging Signs

▶ **Modality of choice**
Function: Echocardiography ● *Morphology and DD:* MRI.

▶ **Chest radiograph findings**
Often normal ● May show a mass distorting the cardiac outline ● Circumscribed enlargement of the cardiac silhouette or cardiomegaly ● Change in pulmonary vascular markings ● May show only nonspecific signs (depending on tumor location and hemodynamic effects) ● May disclose signs of heart failure or congestion ● Pleural or pericardial effusion ● Atelectasis.

▶ **Echocardiographic findings**
Hyperechoic mass ● Irregular margins ● Accurate localization (TEE) ● Possible impairment of cardiac function ● Pericardial effusion (especially with pericardial infiltration).

▶ **CT findings**
Heterogeneous appearance ● Hypodense mass ● Often located in the RA ● Frequent presence of hemorrhagic and necrotic areas ● No calcifications ● Attached to the pericardium ● Infiltration of adjacent vessels or mediastinal organs.

▶ **MRI findings**
Functional and morphologic findings same as echocardiography and CT ● Heterogeneous signal characteristics ● Foci of high T1-weighted signal intensity ● Cauliflower-like appearance.

Clinical Aspects

▶ **Typical presentation**
Cardiac arrhythmias ● Dyspnea ● Possible fever and weight loss ● Other signs of heart failure as a result of tumor location or pericardial effusion ● Pericardial tamponade and right-sided heart failure may develop in extreme cases ● Average interval from symptom onset to diagnosis is approximately 5 months.

▶ **Treatment options**
Many patients require a combination of chemotherapy, radiotherapy, and surgical intervention.

▶ **Course and prognosis**
Poor prognosis ● Metastasis is commonly present at the time of diagnosis.

Fig. 7.13 Histologically confirmed angiosarcoma of the left atrium. Fat-saturated dark-blood T1-weighted TSE sequence after gadolinium-DTPA administration in the four-chamber view shows an enhancing tumor on the lateral atrial wall infiltrating the mitral valve ring (arrow).

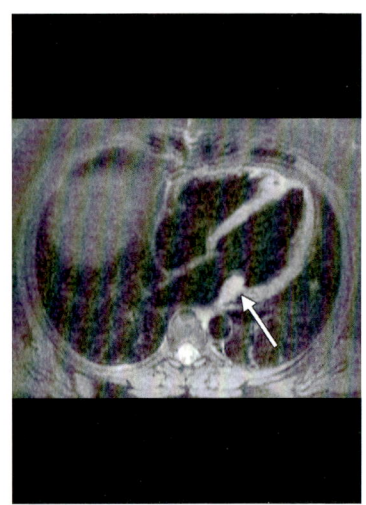

Fig. 7.14 SSFP image at end diastole in the same patient as in Fig. 7.**13**. Recurrent tumor at 4 months appears as a hypointense mass contrasting sharply with the hyperintense blood (arrow). The artifact (*) is the sternal cerclage wires.

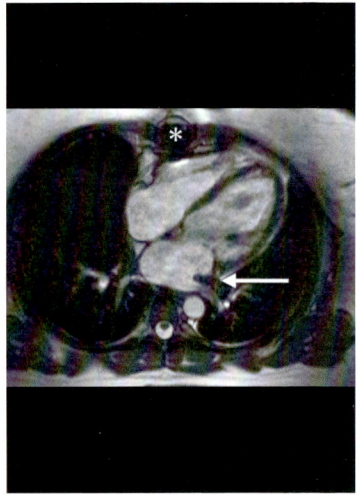

▶ **What does the clinician want to know?**
Precise location and relationships of the tumor (infiltration) ● Impairment of cardiac function ● Pericardial effusion ● Metastases.

Differential Diagnosis

Myxoma	– Often hyperintense on T2-weighted and postcontrast MRI
	– Pedunculated tumor
	– Does not infiltrate surrounding structures
Other masses	– Thrombus
	– Metastasis
	– Other benign or malignant tumors

Tips and Pitfalls

Patients with equivocal Echocardiographic findings require further investigation by MRI.

Selected References

Araoz PA et al. CT and MR imaging of primary cardiac malignancies. RadioGraphics 1999; 19: 1421–1434

Grebenc ML et al. Primary cardiac and pericardial neoplasms: Radiologic-pathologic correlation. Radiographics 2000; 20: 1073–1103

Definition

▶ **Epidemiology**
Synonyms: Pleomorphic sarcoma, round-cell sarcoma, spindle-cell sarcoma • Accounts for less than 24% of all cardiac sarcomas • Average age at diagnosis is 45 years.

▶ **Etiology, pathophysiology, pathogenesis**
No specific histologic markers • Hemorrhagic and necrotic areas • Predilection for the left atrium • May arise from the pericardium • May infiltrate the cardiac valves and other nearby structures • Thrombi sometimes form on the tumor surface.

Imaging Signs

▶ **Modality of choice**
Echocardiography, MRI.

▶ **Chest radiograph findings**
Often normal • May show a mass distorting the cardiac outline • Circumscribed enlargement of the cardiac silhouette or cardiomegaly may be seen • Changes in pulmonary vascular markings • May produce only nonspecific signs (depending on the tumor location and hemodynamic effects) • Heart failure • Signs of congestion • Pleural or pericardial effusion.

▶ **Echocardiographic findings**
Hyperechoic mass in the region of the LA • Irregular margins • Accurate localization (TEE) • Possible impairment of cardiac function (especially mitral valve function) • Pericardial effusion.

▶ **CT findings**
Mass showing a heterogeneous pattern of contrast enhancement • Hemorrhagic and necrotic areas are typical • Thrombi in obstructed vessels (pulmonary veins, vena cava).

▶ **MRI findings**
Functional and morphologic findings same as echocardiography and CT • Heterogeneous signal characteristics • Foci of high T1-weighted signal intensity (hemorrhage) and T2-weighted signal intensity • MRI permits optimum evaluation of the pericardium.

Clinical Aspects

▶ **Typical presentation**
Weight loss • Dyspnea • Chest pain • Heart failure and pulmonary congestion.

▶ **Treatment options**
Appropriate surgical resection increases the survival rate • In rare cases, heart transplantation is available as a last resort.

▶ **Course and prognosis**
Very poor prognosis • Local recurrence is common • Life expectancy of 3–12 months.

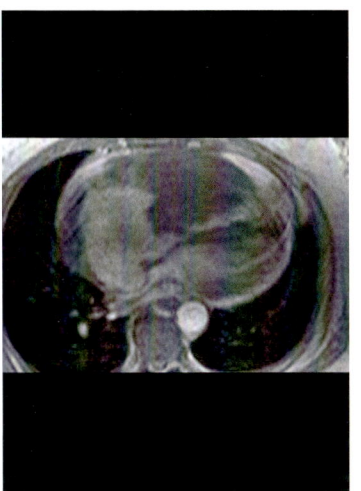

Fig. 7.15 Undifferentiated sarcoma of the right ventricle in a 63-year-old woman. ECG-triggered GRE sequence at end diastole shows an extensive mass in the right ventricle infiltrating the tricuspid valve.

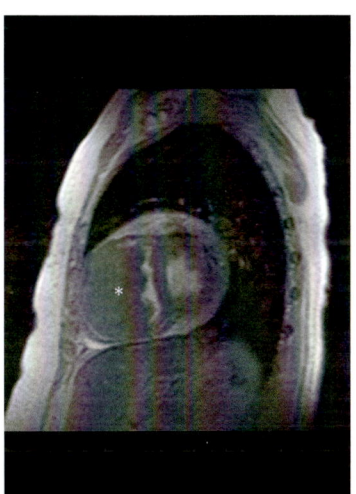

Fig. 7.16 Same patient as in Fig. 7.**15**. ECG-triggered GRE sequence at end diastole shows subtotal occlusion of the right ventricular lumen by the sarcoma (*).

▶ **What does the clinician want to know?**

Precise location and relationships (infiltration) • Impairment of cardiac function • Pericardial effusion • Thrombi.

Differential Diagnosis

Myxoma	– Often hyperintense on T2-weighted and postcontrast MRI
	– Pedunculated tumor
	– Does not infiltrate surrounding structures
Other masses	– Thrombus
	– Metastasis
	– Other malignant cardiac tumors such as angiosarcoma and rhabdomyosarcoma

Tips and Pitfalls

An embolic process may be the earliest sign of a malignant cardiac tumor • Echocardiography is always indicated and may have to be followed by additional studies such as MRI.

Selected References

Colucci WS et al. Primary tumors of the heart. In: Braunwald E. Heart Disease: A Textbook of Cardiovascular Medicine. Philadelphia: Saunders; 2001

Sparrow PJ et al. MR Imaging of Cardiac Tumors. RadioGraphics 2005; 25: 1255–1276

Definition

▶ **Epidemiology**
Very rare tumor • 4–7% of all cardiac sarcomas • Most common malignant cardiac tumor in infants and children • Definite male preponderance.

▶ **Etiology, pathophysiology, pathogenesis**
Originates from striated muscle cells • No predilection for a particular cardiac chamber • Common for multiple masses to arise from the myocardium or cardiac valves • Possible infiltration of the pericardium.

Imaging Signs

▶ **Modality of choice**
Echocardiography.

▶ **Chest radiograph findings**
Often normal • Tumor may distort the cardiac outline • Circumscribed enlargement of the cardiac silhouette or cardiomegaly • Change in pulmonary vascular markings • May show only nonspecific signs (depending on tumor location and hemodynamic effects) • Heart failure • Congestion • Pleural or pericardial effusion.

▶ **Echocardiographic findings**
Iso- to hyperechoic mass • Irregular margins • Accurate localization (TEE) • Evaluation of cardiac function • Pericardial effusion (pericardial infiltration).

▶ **CT findings**
Heterogeneous mass with necrotic areas • Infiltration of the pericardium, adjacent vessels, or mediastinal organs • Possible distant metastases (lung, pleura).

▶ **MRI findings**
Functional and morphologic findings same as echocardiography and CT • Heterogeneous signal characteristics after gadolinium administration • Focal hyperintense areas on T2-weighted images (necrosis).

Clinical Aspects

▶ **Typical presentation**
Variable presentation • Resembles angiosarcoma • Dominant features are signs of heart failure.

▶ **Treatment options**
Tumor resection • Heart transplantation.

▶ **Course and prognosis**
Poor prognosis, due in part to early metastasis • Patients rarely survive longer than 2 years despite treatment.

▶ **What does the clinician want to know?**
Tumor detection • Cardiac function • Infiltration of surrounding structures • Pericardial effusion • Pulmonary metastases.

Differential Diagnosis

Angiosarcoma	– Rhabdomyosarcoma: At least part of the tumor infiltrates the myocardium; nodular pericardial involvement
	– Angiosarcoma: Superficial tumor spread

Tips and Pitfalls

Confusion with myxoma is not uncommon.

Selected References

Araoz PA et al. CT and MR imaging of primary cardiac malignancies. RadioGraphics 1999; 19: 1421–1434

Kosuga T et al. Surgery for primary cardiac tumors. Clinical experience and surgical results in 60 patients. Cardiovasc Surg 2002; 43: 581–587

Sparrow PJ et al. MR imaging of cardiac tumors. RadioGraphics 2005; 25: 1255–1276

Definition

▶ **Epidemiology**
Primary cardiac lymphomas are rarer than cardiac involvement by non-Hodgkin lymphoma (25–36%) ● Increased incidence in immunocompromised patients.

▶ **Etiology, pathophysiology, pathogenesis**
Almost all primary cardiac lymphomas are aggressive B-cell lymphomas ● Pericardial or cardiac involvement ● Predilection for the right heart, especially the right atrium ● Pericardial effusion is common.

Imaging Signs

▶ **Modality of choice**
Echocardiography, MRI (particularly for follow-up).

▶ **Chest radiograph findings**
Enlarged cardiac silhouette due to pericardial effusion ● Additional sites of involvement may be seen (hila, mediastinum, lung) ● Pleural effusion ● Heart failure.

▶ **Echocardiographic findings**
Mass in the pericardium or right heart ● Possible foci of micronodular thickening ● Assessment of cardiac function ● Pericardial effusion.

▶ **CT findings**
Pericardial effusion ● Thickened pericardium ● Single or multiple masses with a inhomogeneous enhancement pattern ● Possible extracardiac manifestations.

▶ **MRI findings**
Same as Echocardiographic and CT findings ● Tumor with low T1-weighted signal intensity ● Inhomogeneous high signal intensity on T2-weighted images and after contrast administration.

▶ **Invasive diagnostic procedures**
For histologic confirmation of the diagnosis ● Pericardiocentesis (aspiration cytology) in patients with pericardial effusion ● *Alternative:* Surgical or interventional biopsy.

Clinical Aspects

▶ **Typical presentation**
Clinical hallmark is rapidly progressive heart failure ● Dyspnea is common ● Signs of pulmonary venous congestion ● Thoracic and epigastric pain ● Occasional arrhythmias ● Obstruction of the superior vena cava ● Pericardial effusion ● Pericardial tamponade.

▶ **Treatment options**
Cardiac lymphomas respond well to early initiation of chemotherapy.

▶ **Course and prognosis**
Generally poor prognosis ● Besides tumor remission (described for 5 years or longer), the severity of heart failure is the most important initial determinant of life expectancy.

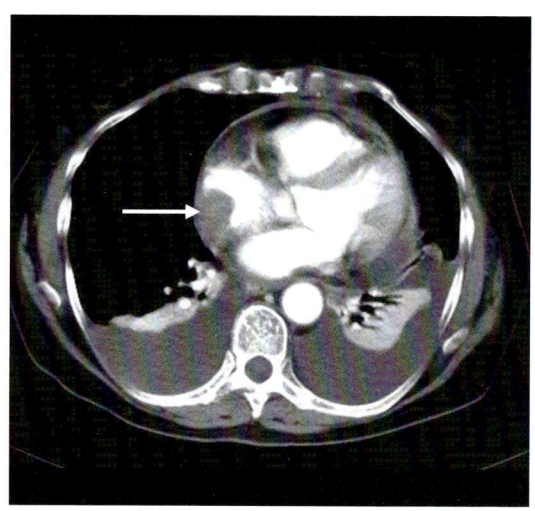

Fig. 7.17 A 60-year-old woman with clinical manifestations of progressive heart failure. Contrast-enhanced axial CT demonstrates a mass on the posterior wall of the RA (arrow) with associated mild pericardial effusion. Cytological examination after pericardiocentesis identified the tumor as B-cell lymphoma. The scan also shows marked bilateral pleural effusion with associated compression atelectasis.

Fig. 7.18 Same patient as in Fig. 7.**17**. Follow-up MR image after two chemotherapy cycles. SSFP image in the four-chamber view documents regression of the mass (arrow) and clearing of the pericardial effusion.

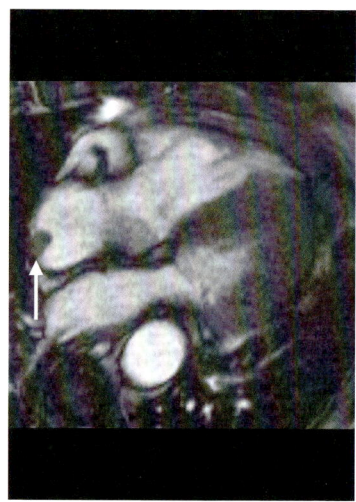

▶ **What does the clinician want to know?**
Detection of a cardiac or pericardial mass ● Pericardial effusion ● Additional sites of occurrence ● Cardiac function ● Signs of right-sided heart failure.

Differential Diagnosis

Cardiac tumors	– Other primary malignant cardiac tumor
	– Extracardiac tumor with pericardial infiltration (pericardial effusion!)
Progressive heart failure	– Pericarditis or myocarditis
	– CHD
	– Cardiomyopathy

Tips and Pitfalls

Diagnostic pericardiocentesis may narrow the DD in patients with unexplained pericardial effusion and progressive heart failure.

Selected References

Kaminaga T et al. Role of magnetic resonance imaging for evaluation of tumors in the cardiac region. Eur Radiol 2003; 13 Suppl 6: L1–L10

Kubo S et al. Primary cardiac lymphoma demonstrated by delayed contrast-enhanced magnetic resonance imaging. J Comput Assist Tomogr 2004; 28: 849–851

Definition

▶ **Epidemiology**
Most of these tumors are leiomyosarcomas ● Average age at diagnosis is approximately 50 years ● Males and females are affected equally.

▶ **Etiology, pathophysiology, pathogenesis**
Usually arises from the pulmonary artery or proximal pulmonary vessels ● May show intravascular growth or may infiltrate surrounding structures.

Imaging Signs

▶ **Modality of choice**
CT.

▶ **Chest radiograph findings**
Often normal ● May demonstrate a hilar mass and mediastinal widening ● Right-heart overload due to pulmonary arterial obstruction ● Congestive signs due to stenosis of pulmonary veins ● Pleural effusion ● Pericardial effusion.

▶ **CT and MRI findings**
Homogeneous intravascular mass ● Sharply circumscribed ● May infiltrate surrounding structures ● Intravascular masses can be distinguished from pulmonary artery embolism by tumor enhancement.

Clinical Aspects

▶ **Typical presentation**
Often asymptomatic ● Possible chest pain ● Dyspnea ● Refractory heart failure ● Hemoptysis.

▶ **Treatment options**
Chemotherapy, radiotherapy, and surgery should be combined whenever possible.

▶ **Course and prognosis**
Poor prognosis ● Average life expectancy is 6–12 months.

▶ **What does the clinician want to know?**
Impairment of cardiac function ● Infiltration of surrounding structures.

Differential Diagnosis

Pulmonary artery embolism – Does not enhance after contrast administration

Selected References

Araoz PA et al. CT and MR imaging of primary cardiac malignancies. RadioGraphics 1999; 19: 1421–1434

Colucci WS et al. Primary tumors of the heart. In: Braunwald E. Heart Disease: A Textbook of Cardiovascular Medicine. Philadelphia: Saunders; 2001

Grebenc ML et al. Primary cardiac and pericardial neoplasms: Radiologic-pathologic correlation. Radiographics 2000; 20(4): 1073–1103

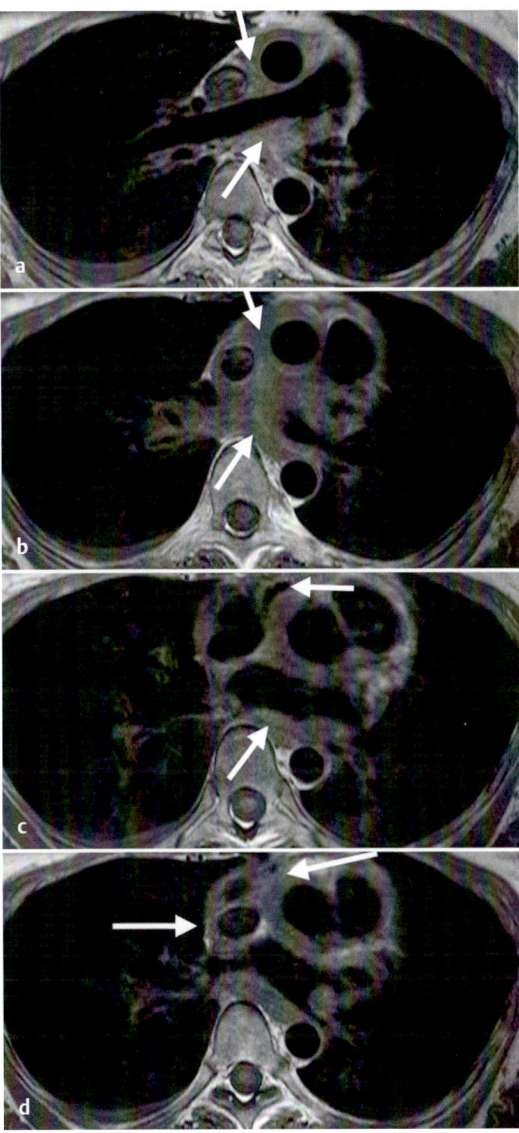

Fig. 7.19 a–d
Recurrence of pulmonary artery sarcoma in a 43-year-old woman. ECG-triggered dark-blood TSE sequence. Axial images show diffuse infiltration of the mediastinum with periaortic and pericardial lesions (arrows).

Definition

▶ **Epidemiology**
Approximately 25–50% of all mediastinal tumors are malignant.
▶ **Etiology, pathophysiology, pathogenesis**
– *Anterior mediastinum:* Goiter • Thyroid tumor • Thymoma (malignant in 50% of cases) • Teratoma (malignant in 30% of cases).
– *Central mediastinum:* Malignant lymphomas • Lymph node metastases • Esophageal carcinoma • Aortic aneurysm.
– *Posterior mediastinum:* Neurofibroma • Neurinoma • Pheochromocytoma • Neuroblastoma.

Imaging Signs

▶ **Modality of choice**
CT.
▶ **Chest radiograph findings**
Broadening of the mediastinum • Displacement and/or compression of surrounding structures (trachea, heart, pleural reflections) • Calcifications (e.g., thymoma, teratoma) • Pleural effusion (especially with pleural involvement).
▶ **Echocardiographic findings**
May be helpful in selected cases for excluding a cardiac tumor or cardiac involvement • Pericardial effusion due to pericardial infiltration.
▶ **CT and MRI findings**
Can accurately define tumor location and extent • Lymph node status •
▶ **PET-CT findings**
Follow-up study of choice in cases with equivocal treatment response • In cases with residual tumor, FDG uptake can be used to assess the viability of tissue remnants in correlation with morphology.

Clinical Aspects

▶ **Typical presentation**
– *Anterior and central mediastinum:* Respiratory distress • Stridor • Dysphagia • Superior vena cava compression.
– *Posterior mediastinum:* Dysphagia • Back pain (compression of intercostal nerves or plexuses).
▶ **Treatment options**
Depend on etiology • Resection, chemotherapy, and/or radiation.
▶ **Course and prognosis**
Depend on tumor type and stage • The rate of remission for stage I–IV Hodgkin disease is over 90% in the first 10 years • The rate of remission for stage I–II NHL is over 88%.

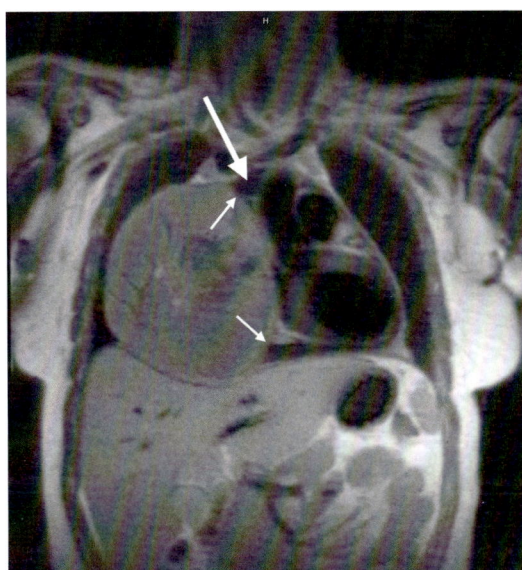

Fig. 7.20 Extensive pericardial mediastinal tumor (identified histologically as a malignant peripheral neuroectodermal tumor). Dark-blood T1-weighted TSE sequence in the coronal plane shows an inhomogeneous mass displacing the heart and compressing the superior vena cava and right atrium (large arrow). The image also shows pericardial effusion secondary to pericardial invasion by the extrapericardial tumor (small arrows = pericardium).

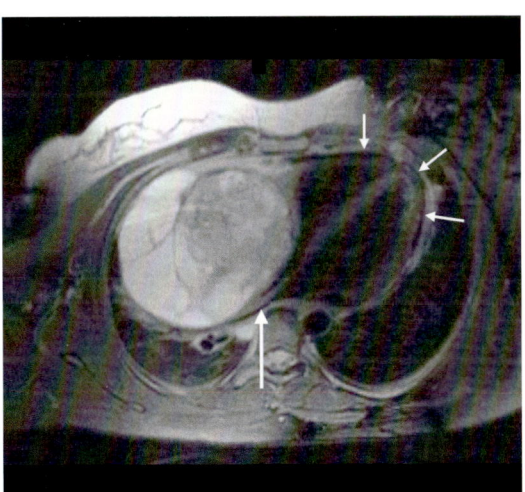

Fig. 7.21 Same patient as in Fig. 7.20. Dark-blood T2-weighted TSE sequence in the four-chamber view shows the hyperintense, septate tumor compressing the RA and the proximal right lower lobe pulmonary vein (large arrow). Pericardial effusion (small arrows) is also seen.

▶ **What does the clinician want to know?**

Location and relations of the tumor • DD • Lymph node status • Infiltration of adjacent structures (heart, vessels) • Impairment of cardiac function • Inflow stasis • Pleural or pericardial effusion.

Differential Diagnosis

Aortic aneurysm, vascular changes	– Can be positively identified by MR- and CT-angiography
Cysts (bronchogenic cyst, pericardial cyst)	– Typical location
	– No contrast enhancement
	– High T2-weighted signal intensity (MRI)
	– Usually show serous attenuation values on CT

Tips and Pitfalls

Devitalized tumor remnants are present in approximately 40% of Hodgkin disease patients in complete remission • Findings should therefore be confirmed by follow-up or PET-CT • With operable tumors, pericardial infiltration is usually a minor consideration whereas infiltration of the cardiac chambers or great vessels is a major concern and may necessitate use of a heart–lung machine.

Selected References

Colucci WS et al. Primary tumors of the heart. In: Braunwald E. Heart Disease: A Textbook of Cardiovascular Medicine. Philadelphia: Saunders; 2001

Schäfer-Prokop C. Mediastinum, pleura and chest wall. From: Prokop M, Galanski M. Spiral and Multislice Computed Tomography of the Body. Stuttgart: Thieme; 2003

Definition

▶ **Epidemiology**
Estimated incidence per year of 0.1% • About more than 10% of fatal complications of motor vehicle accidents are owing to cardiac contusion.

▶ **Pathoanatomy, classification**
Myocardial rupture (LV in most cases, followed by the RV and LA) • Coronary thrombosis • Coronary dissection • Complex arrhythmias due to diffuse myocardial damage • Rupture of the chordae tendineae or papillary muscles (acute myocardial infarction).

▶ **Etiology, pathophysiology, pathogenesis**
Deceleration trauma compresses the heart between the sternum and spinal column (thoracic trauma, resuscitation).

Imaging Signs

▶ **Modality of choice**
Echocardiography.

▶ **Chest radiograph findings**
May show an enlarged cardiac silhouette (pericardial effusion) • Heart failure (pulmonary venous congestion, pleural effusion) • Fractures of the spinal column, sternum, or ribs.

▶ **Echocardiographic findings**
Regional wall motion abnormalities • Muscular defect with hemorrhage (color Doppler) • Pericardial effusion • Mitral insufficiency.

▶ **CT findings**
May reveal a muscular defect or nonenhancing area • Contrast extravasation may result from hemorrhage, pericardial effusion, or a spinal or sternal fracture.

▶ **MRI findings**
Indicated only in the chronic stage • Regional wall motion abnormalities • Possible posttraumatic edema (T2-weighted) • Delayed enhancement of the damaged myocardium after contrast administration.

Clinical Aspects

▶ **Typical presentation**
Symptoms of heart failure or circulatory arrest • Arrhythmias • Chest pain • ECG changes • Elevated CK and troponin.

▶ **Treatment options**
Conservative treatment (surveillance) in hemodynamically stable patients • Severe injuries are treated operatively (ventricular rupture, papillary muscle rupture).

▶ **Course and prognosis**
Mortality is highest (up to 70%) during the acute phase after the trauma • Course and prognosis depend on severity and complications • Spontaneous remission is common and implies good prognosis.

Fig. 8.1 Thoracic trauma sustained in a motor vehicle accident. Supine chest radiograph shows marked broadening of the cardiac silhouette (arrows). The prominent azygos vein indicates right heart overload. The densities in the lower lobes of both lungs are a result of pulmonary contusions and atelectasis. Central venous lines are visible in the superior vena cava.

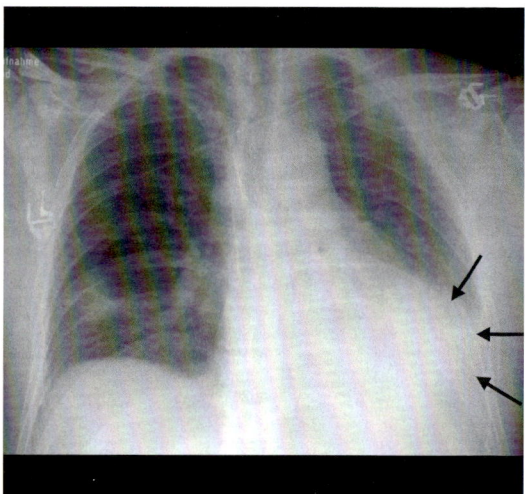

Fig. 8.2 Same patient as in Fig. 8.1. Contrast-enhanced CT shows a circumscribed pericardial hematoma (arrows) resulting from cardiac contusion. There is associated dilatation of the RA and RV.

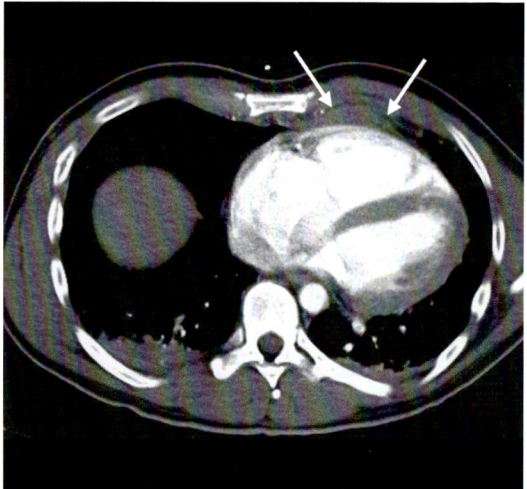

▶ **What does the clinician want to know?**
Ventricular function • Pericardial effusion • Evidence of rupture • Other thoracic injuries.

Differential Diagnosis

Acute trauma	– Aortic dissection or rupture
	– Coronary dissection
	– Myocardial infarction
Subacute stage	– Angina pectoris
	– (Peri)myocarditis
	– Pulmonary embolism
	– Myocardial infarction

Tips and Pitfalls

Cardiac contusion should be considered in patients with severe thoracic trauma, especially sternal and/or vertebral fractures • Possible complications of cardiac contusion should be excluded.

Selected References

Bansal MK et al. Myocardial contusion injury: redefining the diagnostic algorithm. Emerg Med J 2005; 22: 465–469

Mattox KL et al. Traumatic heart disease. In: Braunwald, Zipes, Libby. Heart Disease: A Textbook of Cardiovascular Medicine. Philadelphia: Saunders; 2001

Definition

▶ **Pathoanatomy, classification**
Approximately 70% of ruptures occur in the proximal part of the descending aorta at the origin of the ligamentum arteriosum ● Rare sites of occurrence are the ascending aorta (10%) and thoracoabdominal junction ● A complete (lethal) aortic rupture is distinguished from a confined rupture.

▶ **Etiology, pathophysiology, pathogenesis**
Most common cause is severe thoracic trauma (motor vehicle accident, fall from a great height) ● Violent deceleration ruptures all the layers of the aortic wall.

Imaging Signs

▶ **Modality of choice**
CT.

▶ **Chest radiograph findings**
Mediastinal widening following severe thoracic trauma ● Left hemothorax ● Possible vertebral and rib fractures.

▶ **Echocardiographic findings**
Circumscribed aortic dilatation ● Left hemothorax ● Color Doppler may reveal hemorrhage ● TEE is an option if transthoracic scanning is difficult to carry out.

▶ **CT findings**
With intramural hemorrhage, the aortic wall appears hyperdense on unenhanced scans ● Contrast extravasation occurs at the rupture site, typically at the start of the descending aorta ● Hemopericardium, hemomediastinum, or left hemothorax.

▶ **MRI findings**
MRI is not indicated in this situation.

▶ **Invasive diagnostic procedures**
Angiography is used only in the setting of endovascular therapy.

Clinical Aspects

▶ **Typical presentation**
Most patients present with severe internal injuries ● A small proportion present with specific, stabbing pain between the shoulder blades.

▶ **Treatment options**
Treatment of choice is endoluminal placement of an aortic prosthesis ● Another option is aortic replacement with a tubular prosthesis.

▶ **Course and prognosis**
A complete aortic rupture is instantly fatal ● A confined rupture is acutely life-threatening ● Few patients live long enough to reach the hospital ● Prognosis depends on the intensity of bleeding and the other effects of trauma.

▶ **What does the clinician want to know?**
Site of the rupture (typical location) ● Active bleeding ● Hemothorax and/or hemopericardium ● Mediastinal findings.

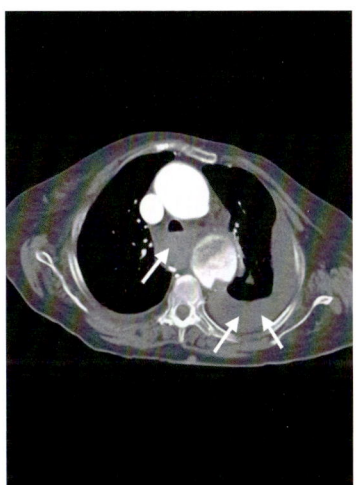

Fig. 8.3   Aortic rupture in a patient with multiple injuries following a motor vehicle accident. Axial postcontrast thoracic multidetector CT shows marked mediastinal widening with a thoracic aortic aneurysm, mediastinal hematoma, and left hemothorax (arrows). The scan shows inhomogeneous opacification of the descending aorta at the rupture site with anterior contrast extravasation.

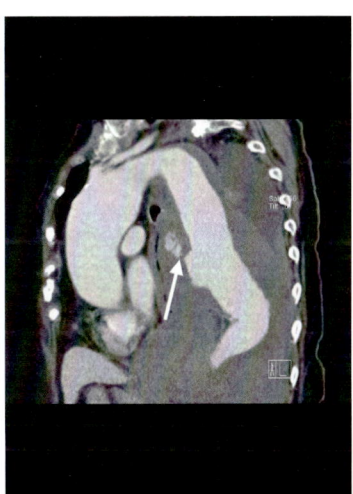

Fig. 8.4   Same patient as in Fig. 8.**3**. Reformatted sagittal image shows anterior contrast extravasation (arrow) and irregular vessel wall contours, signifying active bleeding from the rupture site. Note the extensive periaortic hematoma (density 60 HU).

Differential Diagnosis

Other diseases or injuries of the aorta	– Traumatic aortic dissection
	– Intramural hemorrhage
	– Aortic aneurysm

Tips and Pitfalls

Signs of rupture and bleeding are occasionally subtle (irregular aortic contour, minimal contrast extravasation) • Diagnosis may be aided by three-phase CT: precontrast, arterial, and late phase.

Selected References

Gavant ML et al. Blunt traumatic aortic rupture: detection with helical CT of the chest. Radiology 1995; 197: 125–133

Nzewi O et al. Management of blunt thoracic aortic injury. Eur J Vasc Endovasc Surg 2006; 31: 18–27

Definition

▶ **Epidemiology**
Rare cause of angina pectoris or myocardial infarction.
▶ **Pathoanatomy, classification**
Any coronary territory may be affected, depending on the etiology.
▶ **Etiology, pathophysiology, pathogenesis**
May occur spontaneously in arterial hypertension • Aortic dissection • Postpartum • Giant cell arteritis • Kawasaki syndrome • Iatrogenic cause—catheter or wire intervention • Posttraumatic.

Imaging Signs

▶ **Modality of choice**
Invasive catheter angiography.
▶ **Chest radiograph findings**
No cardiopulmonary abnormalities.
▶ **Echocardiographic findings**
May demonstrate an intimal flap near the ostium (particularly with an aortic dissection).
▶ **CT and MRI findings**
Coronary dissection is not a primary indication for CT or MRI • Dissection may be detected during emergency diagnosis (e.g., thoracic trauma, aortic dissection).
▶ **Invasive diagnostic procedures**
Visualization of the intimal flap by coronary angiography • Evaluation of coronary status • Immediate PTCA or stent implantation may be necessary.

Clinical Aspects

▶ **Typical presentation**
Variable clinical presentation • Some cases are asymptomatic • Possible angina pectoris (acute myocardial infarction) • Sudden cardiac death may occur.
▶ **Treatment options**
Antihypertensive therapy • Anticoagulation • PTCA and/or stent implantation may be indicated.
▶ **Course and prognosis**
Depend on clinical findings • Acute dissection with myocardial infarction has a poor prognosis • Chronic, hemodynamically nonsignificant dissections have a good long-term outcome and often resolve spontaneously.
▶ **What does the clinician want to know?**
Origin and extent of the dissection • Myocardial ischemia • Myocardial infarction • Ventricular function.

Fig. 8.5 Spontaneous coronary dissection in the postpartum period. Coronary angiogram in the RAO projection shows dissection of the left main coronary artery (1) and occlusion of the LAD (2) (from Gasparovic H et al. Surgical treatment of a postpartum spontaneous left main coronary artery dissection. Thorac Cardiovasc Surg 2006; 54; 70–71).

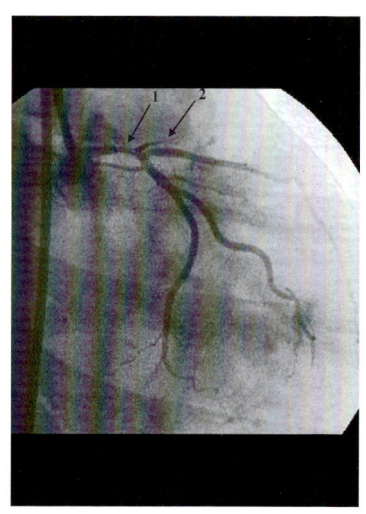

Differential Diagnosis

Coronary heart disease	– Angina pectoris due to CHD
	– Acute myocardial infarction
	– Coronary embolism (plaque, thrombus)
Other thoracic diseases	– Other possible causes of acute chest pain such as (peri)myocarditis, pulmonary embolism, and aortic dissection

Tips and Pitfalls

Coronary dissection may be initially misinterpreted and its hemodynamic effects underestimated (acute myocardial infarction).

Selected References

Gowda RM et al. Clinical perspectives of the primary spontaneous coronary artery dissection. Int J Cardiol 2005; 105: 334–336

Naughton P et al. Spontaneous coronary artery dissection. Emerg Med J 2005; 22: 910–912

Definition

▶ **Epidemiology**
Rare.
▶ **Etiology, pathophysiology, pathogenesis**
Rupture or avulsion of a main pulmonary artery trunk because of severe thoracic trauma • Inflation of a pulmonary artery catheter (Swan–Ganz) may cause vascular injury.

Imaging Signs

▶ **Modality of choice**
CT.
▶ **Chest radiograph findings**
Lung opacity due to intrapulmonary hemorrhage • Pleural effusion due to hemothorax.
▶ **Echocardiographic findings**
May demonstrate the vascular lesion • Active bleeding on TEE (color Doppler).
▶ **CT findings**
Active contrast extravasation in contrast-enhanced CT • Bleeding into the lung parenchyma (ground-glass opacity or complete opacification of a pulmonary segment or lobe) • Hemothorax and/or hemomediastinum.

Clinical Aspects

▶ **Typical presentation**
Usually occurs in the setting of severe thoracic trauma • Hemoptysis • Hypoxemia • Hemodynamic instability due to volume loss.
▶ **Treatment options**
Emergency surgery is the only treatment option in many cases.
▶ **Course and prognosis**
Approximately 50% of cases have a fatal outcome due to rapid circulatory failure and respiratory insufficiency.
▶ **What does the clinician want to know?**
Site of pulmonary artery rupture • Bleeding activity • Intrapulmonary hemorrhage • Hemothorax • Associated injuries • Position of a flow-directed catheter, if present.

Fig. 8.6 Woman who sustained multiple injuries in a motor vehicle accident. Axial postcontrast multidetector CT shows bilateral pneumothorax, hyperdense areas of intrapulmonary hemorrhage (small arrows), and left hemothorax (large arrow). Suspicion of pulmonary artery rupture was confirmed at operation.

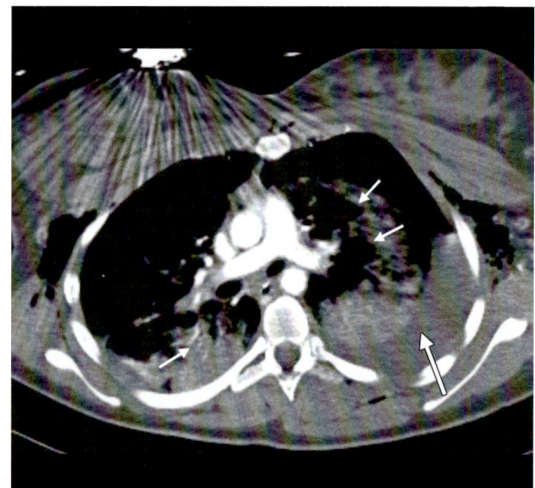

Fig. 8.7 Same patient as in Fig. 8.**6**. Reformatted coronal image shows increased density in the left lung due partly to intrapulmonary hemorrhage and partly to contusions (arrows). Other findings are bilateral pneumothorax and pronounced emphysema of the chest wall (*). An endotracheal tube is also visible. The very narrow vessels and small heart are the result of circulatory shock and significant blood loss.

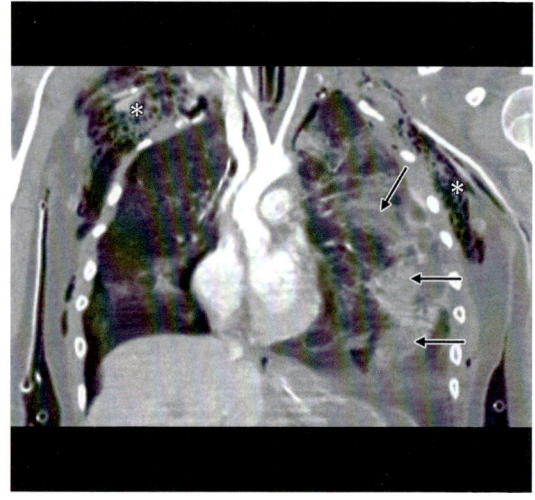

Differential Diagnosis

Trauma	– Injury of a cardiac chamber (ventricular rupture) or major thoracic vessel (aorta, subclavian artery)
Other	– Pulmonary embolism with acute onset of right-sided heart failure, dyspnea, and/or tachypnea
	– Hemoptysis due to other causes (e.g., tumor, pulmonary infarction, Wegener granulomatosis, Behçet disease)

Tips and Pitfalls

Consider a pulmonary artery rupture or pseudoaneurysm in patients with a pulmonary artery catheter (Swan–Ganz) and new pulmonary opacities.

Selected References

Abreu AR et al. Pulmonary artery rupture induced by a pulmonary artery catheter: a case report and review of the literature. J Intensive Care Med 2004; 19: 291–296

Choong CK, Meyers BF. Lung mass after pulmonary artery catheterization: beware of the pulmonary artery false aneurysm. J Thorac Cardiovasc Surg 2005; 130: 899–900

Definition

▶ **Epidemiology**

Isolated ASD accounts for 5–10% of all cardiac anomalies • More common in females than in males (2:1) • A third of all congenital heart defects are not diagnosed until adulthood.

▶ **Etiology, pathophysiology, pathogenesis**

Up to 40% of small ASDs may close spontaneously by the age of 5 years • Extent and direction of the shunt depend on the size of the defect and the compliance of the ventricles • ASDs smaller than 0.5 cm are not hemodynamically significant • Defects larger than 2 cm produce a hemodynamically significant shunt • Approximately 10% of patients with a hemodynamically significant shunt will develop pulmonary hypertension • Reversal to a right-to-left shunt (Eisenmenger syndrome) occurs in extreme cases.

▶ **Pathoanatomy**

Ostium primum defect (15% of all ASDs) • Ostium secundum defect; special form—patent foramen ovale (75%) • Sinus venosus defect (approximately 10%) • Coronary sinus defect (rare).

Imaging Signs

▶ **Modality of choice**

Echocardiography.

▶ **Chest radiograph and CT findings**

Prominent pulmonary vessels due to the recirculating blood volume • RV enlargement due to volume overload • Late stage is marked by interstitial lung changes • Not a primary indication for CT.

▶ **Echocardiographic findings**

Enlargement of the RA and RV • Enlarged pulmonary arteries with accelerated flow through the pulmonary valve • Assessment of pulmonary arterial pressures • Visualization and quantification of the shunt by color Doppler • Evaluation may be aided with an ultrasound contrast agent.

▶ **MRI findings**

Indicated only if associated cardiac anomalies are suspected • Same as echocardiographic findings • Visualization of anatomy • Evaluation of cardiac function • The shunt can be quantified by comparing the stroke volumes or by flowmetry (comparative flow measurements of pulmonary and systemic flow [Q_p:Q]$_s$.

▶ **Invasive diagnostic procedures**

Rarely necessary during the initial workup • Coronary angiography may be done to exclude a coronary anomaly (multidetector CT can also be used) or CHD in adults • Invasive quantification of shunt flow • ASD may be correctible by implanting an occluder system.

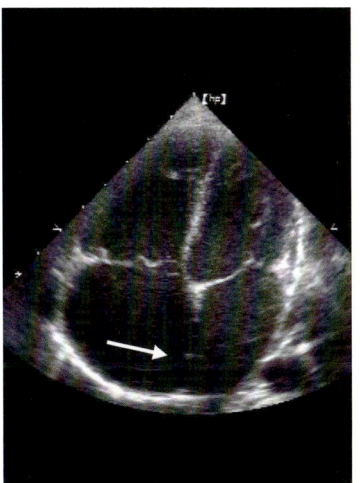

Fig. 9.1 Atrial septal defect (ASD). Four-chamber view (echocardiography) shows a broad defect (arrow) in the interatrial septum (with kind permission of L. Sieverding and G. Greil, Tübingen).

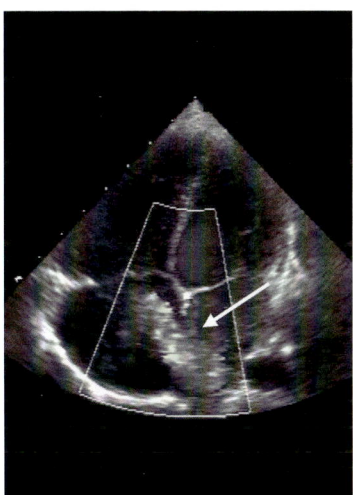

Fig. 9.2 Color Doppler echocardiography in the same patient as in Fig. 9.**1**. Four-chamber view shows a left-to-right shunt (arrow) in the area of the defect (with kind permission of L. Sieverding and G. Greil, Tübingen).

Clinical Aspects

▶ **Typical presentation**

Decreased exercise tolerance • Delayed physical development • Dyspnea on exertion • More frequent bronchopulmonary infections • Patients over 30 years of age present with atrial arrhythmias, right-sided heart failure, paradoxical emboli.

▶ **Treatment options**

An ASD with $Q_p:Q_s$ > 2:1 should be occluded before 5 years of age if at all possible (caution in cases where pulmonary hypertension has already developed) • Defect can be closed by direct suture or patched through a sternotomy • Alternative method is interventional closure (with defect < 38 mm and 5–6 mm of residual septum inferiorly and superiorly) • Postinterventional aspirin regimen (2 mg/kg body weight per day) for 6 months • Endocarditis prophylaxis for several months.

▶ **Course and prognosis**

If the ASD remains patent, 5–10% of patients will develop pulmonary hypertension by 20 years of age • Overt heart failure usually does not develop before 40 years • More than half of patients over 60 years have atrial fibrillation • ASD closure before 6 years implies a good prognosis with no significant reduction in life expectancy.

▶ **What does the clinician want to know?**

Size and location of the ASD • Quantification of the shunt ($Q_p:Q_s$ > 1.5) • Coexisting anomalies • Signs of pulmonary hypertension.

Differential Diagnosis

PDA	– All intracardiac defects with abnormal shunting of blood lead to decreased aortic flow
	– PDA: Prominent aorta
Heart failure in general	– Cardiomyopathies
	– Arrhythmias
	– CHD

Tips and Pitfalls

It is too late for an ASD repair after irreversible pulmonary arterial changes (fixed pulmonary hypertension) have developed. • *Caution:* Do not overlook more complex anomalies such as ASD with a VSD or AVSD.

Selected References

McDaniel NL. Ventricular and atrial septal defects. Pediatr Rev 2001; 22: 265–270
Moake L, Ramaciotti C. Atrial septal defect treatment options. AACN Clin Issues 2005; 16: 252–266

Definition

▶ **Epidemiology**

Most common congenital cardiac anomaly (15–30%) • Approximately 50% of VSD patients have associated anomalies • Up to 40% of VSDs close spontaneously during the first year of life.

▶ **Etiology, pathophysiology, pathogenesis**

The degree and direction of the shunt depend on the size of the septal defect and the ratio of the pulmonary and systemic vascular resistance (primary left-to-right shunt) • Small defects can maintain a pressure gradient • Shunt reversal may occur due to rising pressures in the pulmonary vasculature (Eisenmenger syndrome).

▶ **Pathoanatomy**

The septal defect may be located at various sites:
– Membranous septum (perimembranous VSD, 70%).
– Trabecular septum (muscular VSD, 20%).
– Infundibular septum (5–7%).
– Inlet septum (5–8%).

Imaging Signs

▶ **Modality of choice**

Echocardiography

▶ **Chest radiograph findings**

Cardiomegaly • Prominent pulmonary vessels due to the recirculating blood volume • Enlargement of the right heart and LA due to volume overload • Not a primary indication for CT.

▶ **Echocardiographic findings**

Size and location of the defect • Direction and pressure gradient of the shunt • Assessment of pulmonary arterial pressures • Associated defects and anomalies (e.g., secondary aortic insufficiency) • Dilatation of the LV and LA.

▶ **MRI findings**

Indicated only if associated cardiac anomalies are suspected • Same as echocardiographic findings • Visualization of anatomy • Cardiac function • The shunt can be quantified by comparing the stroke volumes or by flowmetry (see also ASD, page 188).

▶ **Invasive diagnostic procedures**

Rarely necessary during the initial workup • Coronary angiography may be done to exclude a coronary anomaly (multidetector CT can also be used) or CHD in adults • Invasive quantification of shunt flow.

Fig. 9.3 Ventricular septal defect. P-A chest radiograph shows biventricular enlargement of the heart and prominent pulmonary vessels (arrow) due to pulmonary recirculation.

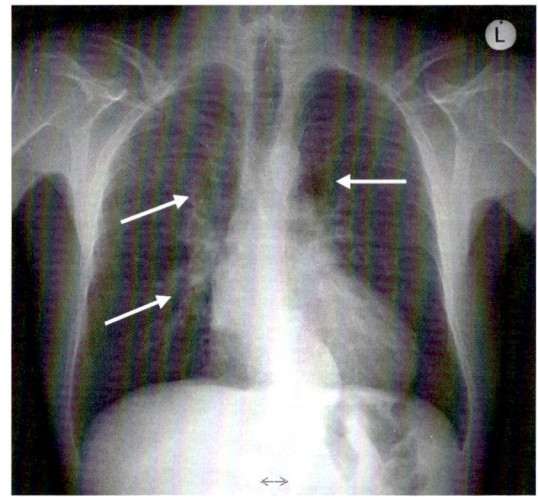

Fig. 9.4 a, b Same patient as in Fig. 9.**3**. Echocardiography (**a**) and color Doppler (**b**) in the four-chamber view demonstrate a VSD (arrow) with a left-to-right shunt (with kind permission of L. Sieverding and G. Greil, Tübingen).

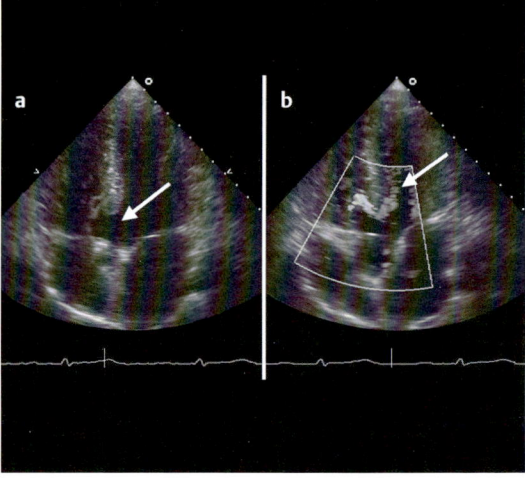

Clinical Aspects

▶ **Typical presentation**
Children:. Sweating • Respiratory distress • Bronchopulmonary infections • As pressure rises in the pulmonary circulation, symptoms regress • Shunt reversal leads to cyanosis • Small defects are usually asymptomatic.
Adults: Pulmonary hypertension leading to heart failure • Atrial fibrillation • Paradoxical emboli (TIA, stroke).

▶ **Treatment options**
Medical therapy of overt heart failure • Endocarditis prophylaxis in exposed patients • Surgical closure in cases with Q_p:Q_s > 2:1, systolic pulmonary arterial pressure > 50 mmHg, or severe heart failure (*Caution:* Apply rigorous selection criteria in pulmonary hypertension) • Surgery is usually done at 3–9 months of age.

▶ **Course and prognosis**
Without surgery: Small VSDs often close spontaneously during the first 2 years of life, with a very good prognosis • Medium-sized and large VSDs may lead to heart failure and pulmonary hypertension.
After surgery: Good prognosis in patients with normal postoperative ventricular function • Prolonged volume overload may lead to atrial fibrillation • Ventricular arrhythmias • Third-degree AV block (< 5%) • Significant residual VSD in 2–10% of cases.

▶ **What does the clinician want to know?**
Size and location of the VSD • Quantification of the shunt (Q_p:Q_s > 1.5) • Associated aortic insufficiency • Possible coexisting anomalies • Signs of pulmonary hypertension.

Differential Diagnosis

PDA	– All intracardiac defects with abnormal shunting of blood lead to decreased aortic flow
	– PDA: Prominent aorta
Heart failure	– Cardiomyopathies
	– Arrhythmias
	– CHD

Tips and Pitfalls

It is too late for a VSD repair after irreversible pulmonary arterial changes (fixed pulmonary hypertension) have developed. • *Caution:* Rule out the presence of multiple VSDs.

Selected References
Otterstad JE et al. Doppler echocardiography in adults with isolated ventricular septal defect. Eur Heart J 1984; 5: 332–337
Stauder NI et al. MRI diagnosis of a previously undiagnosed large trabecular ventricular septal defect in an adult after multiple catheterizations and angiocardiograms. Br J Radiol 2001; 74: 280–282

Definition

▶ **Definition, pathophysiology, pathogenesis**
Obstructive disease of the pulmonary vasculature based on a pronounced left-to-right shunt of long duration ● When pulmonary arterial resistance reaches the level of the systemic circulation, shunt reversal occurs with a bidirectional or right-to-left shunt.

Imaging Signs

▶ **Modality of choice**
Shunt can be detected and quantified by color Doppler or invasive pressure measurement ● MRI in the evaluation stage.

Clinical Aspects

▶ **Typical presentation**
Severe symptoms often first appear in adolescents and adults ● Progressive dyspnea and cyanosis ● Decreased exercise tolerance ● Severe heart failure ● Angina pectoris ● Paradoxical emboli ● Arrhythmia (atrial fibrillation) ● Infectious endocarditis.

▶ **Treatment options**
Specific treatment is not an option in most cases ● Restrictions on physical activity ● Medical therapy for heart failure ● Oxygen therapy for cyanosis ● Treatment of infections ● Heart–lung transplantation is an option in rare cases (10-year survival rate < 30%) ● Pulmonary vascular resistance can be lowered by CO_2 inhalation and, if necessary, prostaglandin infusion.

▶ **Course and prognosis**
Forty-two percent of patients with Eisenmenger syndrome reach 25 years of age ● Leading causes of death are sudden cardiac death (30%), heart failure (25%), and hemoptysis (15%).

▶ **What does the clinician want to know?**
Signs of increased RV pressure ● Signs of pulmonary hypertension ● Shunt detection ● Features of the underlying cardiac anomaly ● Pulmonary status.

Differential Diagnosis

Other anomalies	– Cyanotic heart disease without Eisenmenger syndrome
Dyspnea or heart failure due to other causes	– Cardiac arrhythmias – Pneumonia

Selected References

Brickner ME, Hillis LD, Lange RA. Congenital heart disease in adults: second of two parts. N Engl J Med 2000; 342(5): 334–342

Hopkins WE. The remarkable right ventricle of patients with Eisenmenger syndrome. Coron Artery Dis 2005; 16: 19–25

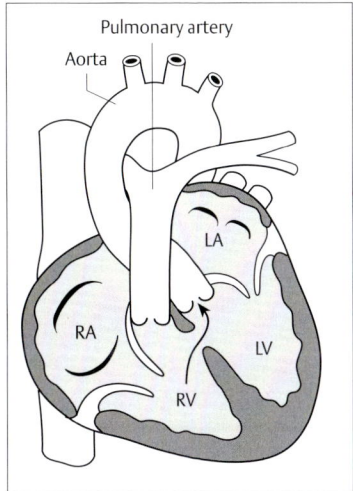

Fig. 9.5 Eisenmenger syndrome. Changes in the small pulmonary arteries and arterioles (media hypertrophy, intimal proliferation and fibrosis) lead to increased resistance in the pulmonary circulation, causing a reversal of the shunt (e.g., with an accompanying VSD, arrow).

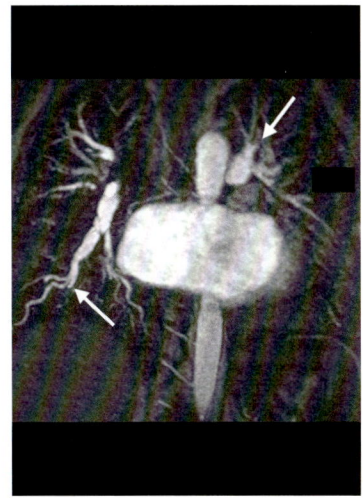

Fig. 9.6 Eisenmenger syndrome in a patient with pulmonary hypertension. Coronal MIP image from a contrast-enhanced MR angiographic study shows an abrupt caliber change between the central and peripheral pulmonary arteries (arrow).

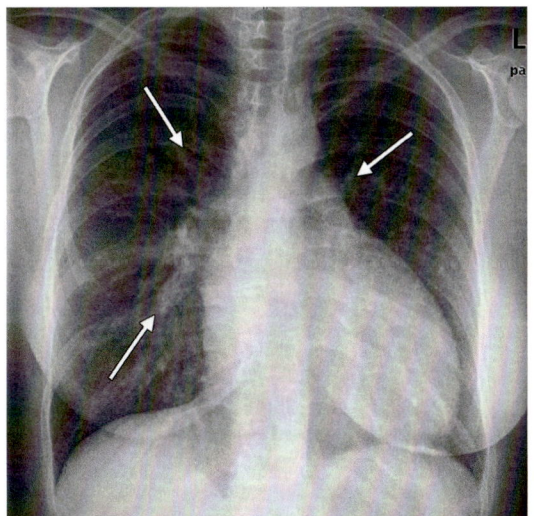

Fig. 9.7 Chest radiograph in the same patient as in Fig. 9.6 shows rapid tapering from the central to peripheral pulmonary arteries (arrow).

Definition

▶ **Epidemiology**
Accounts for 5–10% of all congenital cardiac anomalies • Higher incidence in premature infants • More common in males than in females (3:1) • PDA may be life-saving in the presence of complex anomalies such as HLHS, dextro-TGA, or pulmonary atresia.

▶ **Pathoanatomy**
Fetal vascular connection between the bifurcation of the pulmonary artery and the descending aorta • Generally closes on the first day of life (or during the first 3 weeks in premature infants).

▶ **Etiology, pathophysiology, pathogenesis**
Systolic–diastolic left-to-right shunt • Volume overload on the LA, LV, aortic root, and pulmonary vessels.

Imaging Signs

▶ **Modality of choice**
Echocardiography.

▶ **Chest radiograph findings**
Cardiomegaly due to LA and LV dilatation • Increased diameter of the pulmonary vessels and aortic arch due to the shunt.

▶ **Echocardiographic findings**
Direct visualization of the PDA • Diameter • Direction of the shunt • Pressure gradient • Diastolic flow • Exclusion of other cardiac anomalies.

▶ **MRI findings**
Same as echocardiographic findings • Estimation of shunt volume with flowmetry.

▶ **Invasive diagnostic procedures**
Necessary only in patients with associated complex cyanotic heart disease.

Clinical Aspects

▶ **Typical presentation**
Heart failure • Dyspnea • Atrial arrhythmias • Bronchopulmonary infections.

▶ **Treatment options**
Indometacin is effective treatment for PDA closure only in premature infants • Endocarditis prophylaxis in exposed patients • Surgical or interventional closure is indicated due to the high risk of endocarditis (*Caution:* Established pulmonary hypertension) • PDAs smaller than 6 mm can be closed by the interventional placement of coils or an occlusion system.

▶ **Course and prognosis**
Interventional closure has a primary success rate of 85%, surgical closure > 95% (mortality < 1%).

▶ **What does the clinician want to know?**
Detection of the PDA • Exclusion of other congenital anomalies • Quantification of the shunt volume.

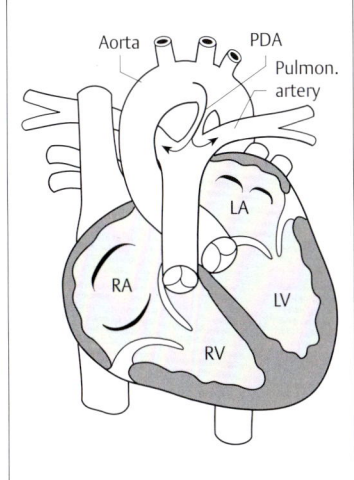

Fig. 9.8 PDA with a left-to-right shunt. Note the dilatation of the left atrium and ventricle.

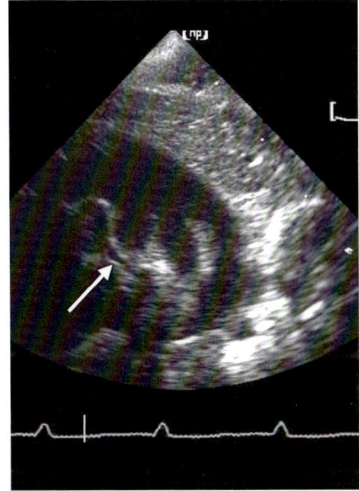

Fig. 9.9 PDA. Echocardiography displays the communication between the aorta and pulmonary artery (arrow) (with kind permission of L. Sieverding, Tübingen).

Differential Diagnosis

Persistent fetal circulation syndrome	– Pulmonary hypertension (due to lung disease)
	– PFO
	– PDA caused by marked hypoxia

Tips and Pitfalls

Do not miss the optimum timing for surgical or interventional treatment. Once severe obstructive changes have developed in the pulmonary vessels, repair of the PDA becomes problematic.

Selected References

Hermes-DeSantis ER, Clyman RI. Patent ductus arteriosus: pathophysiology and management. J Perinatol 2006; 26 Suppl 1:S14–S18; discussion S22–S33

Schneider DJ, Moore JW. Patent ductus arteriosus. Circulation 2006; 114: 1873–1882

Swartz EN. Is indomethacin or ibuprofen better for medical closure of the patent ductus arteriosus? Arch Dis Child 2003; 88: 1134–1135

Wang ZJ et al. Cardiovascular shunts: MR imaging evaluation. Radiographics 2003; 23 Spec No: S181–S194

Wyllie J. Treatment of patent ductus arteriosus. Semin Neonatol 2003; 8: 425–432

Definition

▶ **Epidemiology**
Most common congenital malformation of the aortic valve (prevalence 2%) • Increased incidence of aortic dissection • Often associated with coarctation of the aorta and Marfan syndrome • More common in males than in females (4:1).

▶ **Pathoanatomy**
The aortic valve has two cusps instead of three, substantially increasing the mechanical load • Most frequent manifestation in infants is stenosis • Valvular insufficiency is more common in young adults and atherosclerotic stenosis in older patients.

Imaging Signs

▶ **Modality of choice**
Echocardiography.

▶ **Chest radiograph findings**
Normal in patients with a functioning aortic valve • Possible signs of aortic stenosis or insufficiency.

▶ **Echocardiographic findings**
Aortic valve with two cusps • May detect aortic stenosis or insufficiency, which can be quantified by color Doppler • Evaluation of LV function • Possible association with other anomalies (e.g., coarctation of the aorta).

▶ **MRI findings**
Same as echocardiographic findings • Can more accurately quantify the regurgitant fraction (by phase-contrast imaging) • Better than echocardiography for detecting malformations of the great vessels (MRA).

▶ **Invasive diagnostic procedures**
Older patients should undergo preoperative coronary angiography to exclude CHD.

Clinical Aspects

▶ **Typical presentation**
Often asymptomatic in younger patients • Aortic stenosis or insufficiency develops by 40–60 years of age.

▶ **Treatment options**
Aortic valve replacement for significant valvular dysfunction.

▶ **Course and prognosis**
Predisposes to premature aortic valve degeneration and vegetations in the setting of endocarditis • Endocarditis prophylaxis needed before procedures that may cause bacteremia (e.g., dental procedures, endoscopy).

▶ **What does the clinician want to know?**
Functional impairment (insufficiency, stenosis) • Hemodynamic quantification.

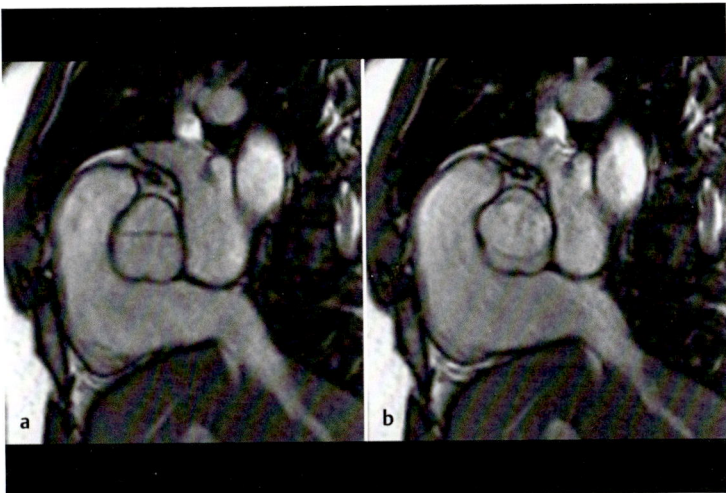

Fig. 9.10 a, b Bicuspid aortic valve. SSFP image parallel to the aortic valve plane shows two valve cusps in the closed position (diastole, **a**) and open position (systole, **b**).

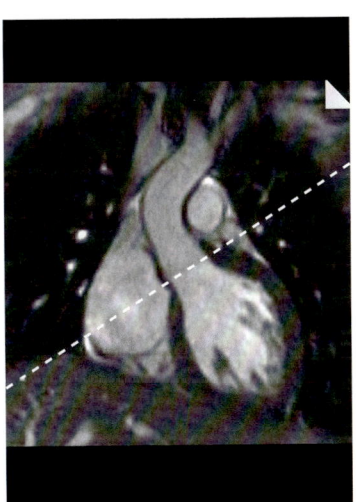

Fig. 9.11 SSFP image of the LVOT. The dashed line indicates the level of the short-axis slice parallel to the valvular plane.

Differential Diagnosis

Degenerative aortic stenosis	– Atherogenic risk factors – Calcification of the valve
Rheumatic changes in the aortic valve	– Fusion of the commissures with fibrosis and thickening of the valve leaflets – Almost always combined with rheumatic mitral valve disease

Tips and Pitfalls

A bicuspid aortic valve should always be considered in patients with coarctation of the aorta because of their association, and the aortic valve should be examined accordingly (by echocardiography).

Selected References

Aboulhosn J, Child JS. Left ventricular outflow obstruction: subaortic stenosis, bicuspid aortic valve, supravalvar aortic stenosis, and coarctation of the aorta. Circulation 2006; 114: 2412–2422

Borth-Bruns T, Eichler A (eds.). Pädiatrische Kardiologie. Berlin, Heidelberg: Springer; 2004

Braverman AC et al. The bicuspid aortic valve. Curr Probl Cardiol 2005; 30: 470–522

Kumpf M, Borth-Bruns T, Nollert G. Angeborene Herzfehler. In: Mewis C, Riessen R, Spyridopoulos I (eds.). Kardiologie compact. Stuttgart: Thieme; 2004

Rigatelli G, Rigatelli G. Congenital heart diseases in aged patients: clinical features, diagnosis, and therapeutic indications based on the analysis of a twenty five-year Medline search. Cardiol Rev 2005; 13: 293–296

Zeppilli P et al. Bicuspid aortic valve: an innocent finding or a potentially life-threatening anomaly whose complications may be elicited by sports activity? J Cardiovasc Med 2006; 7: 282–287

Definition

▶ **Epidemiology**
Comprises 7% of all congenital cardiac anomalies • More common in males than in females (1.5:1) • Incidence of 35% in Turner syndrome.

▶ **Pathoanatomy**
Discrete, membrane–like stenosis located distal to the origin of the left subclavian artery at the ligamentum arteriosum • 50% of patients have isolated coarctation of the aorta with or without a PDA and collateral vessels • Another 50% have associated cardiovascular anomalies.

▶ **Etiology, pathophysiology, pathogenesis**
Arterial hypertension in the upper half of the body • Pressure more than 20 mmHg lower in the lower half of the body • Hypertension is usually present due to decreased renal blood flow.

Imaging Signs

▶ **Modality of choice**
Echocardiography for initial diagnosis • MRI for follow-up in older patients.

▶ **Chest radiograph and CT findings**
Indirect signs of LV hypertrophy • Notching of the ribs • "Figure 3" sign may demonstrate the coarctation itself (this can always be done with CTA) • Strong indication for CT, especially for early posttherapeutic follow-up.

▶ **Echocardiographic and MRI findings**
Location and extent of the coarctation • Associated anomalies • Assessment of pressure gradient by color Doppler (echocardiography) or flow measurement (phase-contrast imaging, MRI) • Blood jet indicates the obstructive effect of the stenosis • Aortic insufficiency (higher incidence of bicuspid aortic valve).

▶ **Invasive diagnostic procedures**
Indicated only in selected cases, e.g., for invasive measurement of the pressure gradient or in the setting of interventional treatment • Coronary angiography.

Clinical Aspects

▶ **Typical presentation**
Often asymptomatic • Symptoms of arterial hypertension (headache, vertigo, epistaxis, palpitations) • Patients over 40 years of age often manifest heart failure • Hypertension in the upper half of the body • Absent or diminished femoral pulses.

▶ **Treatment options**
Open or interventional correction is indicated in patients with a systolic resting pressure gradient > 20–30 mmHg, more than 50% luminal narrowing, marked collateralization, or a rising pressure gradient during exercise • The treatment of choice for newborns and infants is surgical resection of the coarcted segment followed by end-to-end anastomosis (surgical mortality 1–1.4%) • Some patients may require interposition of a vascular prosthesis • Percutaneous balloon

Fig. 9.12 An isolated coarctation of the aorta (CoA) distal to the left subclavian artery. Left ventricular myocardial hypertrophy has resulted from the pressure load on the LV.

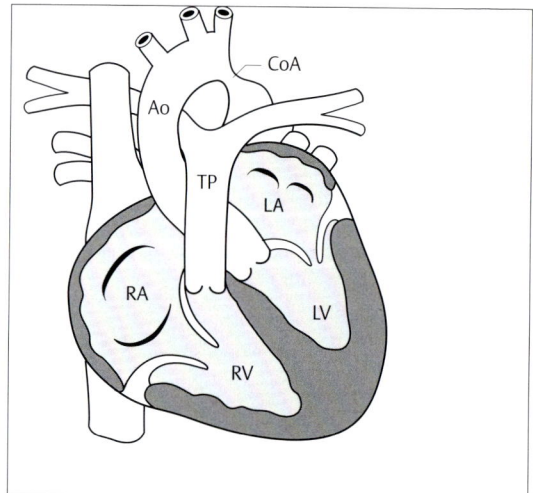

Fig. 9.13 Coarctation of the aorta in a 5-year-old boy. MR angiographic image, oblique sagittal MIP demonstrates a coarctation distal to the origin of the supraaortic vessels (arrows).

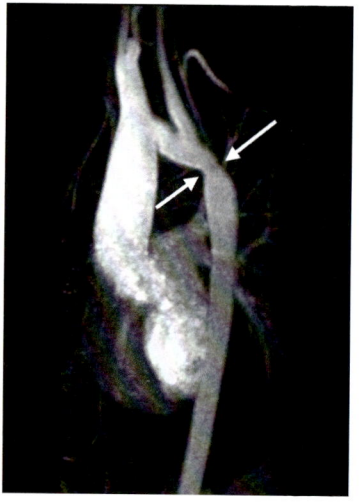

dilatation is an option in adults and for recurrent stenosis (complications are rupture, aneurysm formation, dissection).

Aftercare: Postoperative endocarditis prophylaxis for at least 6 months • Follow-up to exclude restenosis or aneurysm formation • Postoperative paradoxical rebound hypertension (β-blocker therapy).

▶ **Course and prognosis**

Life expectancy is approximately 35 years without treatment, with 90% mortality by 60 years • Main causes of death are left-sided heart failure (28%), aortic rupture or dissection (21%), endocarditis (18%), intracranial hemorrhage (12%), and incompetence of the often bicuspid aortic valve.

▶ **What does the clinician want to know?**

Vascular diameter at the coarctation site • Pressure gradient • Collateral vessels • Associated cardiac anomalies (e.g., bicuspid aortic valve, VSD).

Differential Diagnosis

HLHS	– Hypoplastic LV
	– Heart failure in newborns
	– Ductal-dependent systemic perfusion
	– Retrograde flow in the hypoplastic ascending aorta
Interrupted aortic arch	– Descending aorta perfused through a PDA
Pseudocoarctation of the aorta	– Elongation and kinking of the aorta without stenosis

Tips and Pitfalls

Coarctation of the aorta frequently coexists with other anomalies, and this possibility should be investigated by imaging studies. Associated anomalies include aortic arch hypoplasia, anomalies of the head and neck vessels (aberrant right subclavian artery, 5%), a bicuspid aortic valve (up to 85%), mitral valve anomalies, and VSD.

Selected References

de Divitiis M et al. Arterial hypertension and cardiovascular prognosis after successful repair of aortic coarctation: a clinical model for the study of vascular function. Nutr Metab Cardiovasc Dis 2005; 1: 382–394

Golden AB, Hellenbrand WE. Coarctation of the aorta: stenting in children and adults. Catheter Cardiovasc Interv 2007; 69: 289–299

Kumpf M, Borth-Bruns T, Nollert G. Angeborene Herzfehler. In: Mewls C, Riessen R, Spyridopoulos I (eds.). Kardiologie compact. Stuttgart: Thieme; 2004

Rao PS. Coarctation of the aorta. Curr Cardiol Rep 2005; 7: 425–434

Sebastia C et al. Aortic stenosis: spectrum of diseases depicted at multisection CT. Radiographics 2003; 23 Spec No: S79–S91

Shih MC et al. Surgical and endovascular repair of aortic coarctation: normal findings and appearance of complications on CT angiography and MR angiography. AJR Am J Roentgenol 2006; 187: W302–W312

Vriend JW, Mulder BJ. Late complications in patients after repair of aortic coarctation: implications for management. Int J Cardiol 2005; 101: 399–406

Definition

▶ **Epidemiology**
- Double aortic arch (DAo): Most common vascular ring anomaly (40–55%) ●
  Rarely accompanied by other anomalies.
- Retroesophageal right aortic arch (RAo, 30%): Present in 25% of patients with
  TOF and in 30–40% of patients with truncus arteriosus.

▶ **Etiology, pathoanatomy**
Anomalous persistence of the fourth pharyngeal arch artery, exerting pressure
on the trachea, esophagus, or both (less common with right aortic arch).

Imaging Signs

▶ **Modality of choice**
Echocardiography in small children, MRI in adults

▶ **Chest radiograph findings**
- *DAo:* Soft-tissue densities on both side of the trachea ● Bilateral tracheal narrowing.
- *RAo:* Soft-tissue density to the right of the trachea ● Tracheal narrowing or
  displacement on the right side.

▶ **Barium swallow findings**
A-P projection shows bilateral narrowing of the esophagus at different levels ●
Lateral projection shows marked posterior narrowing of the esophagus.

▶ **Echocardiographic findings**
Two separate aortic arches, each giving rise to a carotid and subclavian artery.

▶ **CT and MRI findings**
Can demonstrate the duplicated or right-sided aortic arch ● Right arch is often
larger (75%) ● Right arch often is located posterosuperiorly and often runs be-
hind the esophagus.

Clinical Aspects

▶ **Typical presentation**
- *DAo:* Stidor and respiratory distress are often present in newborns ● Symp-
  toms are exacerbated by feeding.
- *RAo:* Often asymptomatic ● Increased incidence of pulmonary infections ●
  Stridor.

▶ **Treatment options**
- *DAo:* Thoracotomy with division of the smaller aortic arch.
- *RAo:* May be correctible by aortopexy ● Division of a symptomatic ligamen-
  tum arteriosum.

▶ **Course and prognosis**
Up to 30% of patients have persistent symptoms due to respiratory tract obstruction or compression ● Tracheomalacia ● Some cases may require reoperation
with aortopexy ● Prognosis depends on associated anomalies.

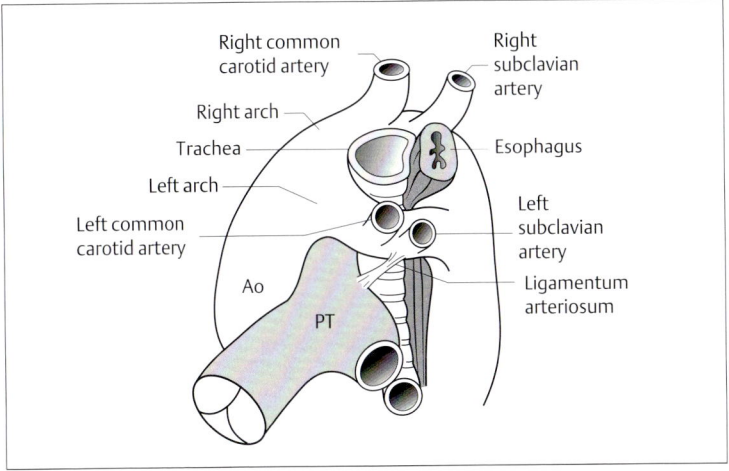

Fig. 9.14 Diagrammatic illustration of a double aortic arch with a dominant right arch.

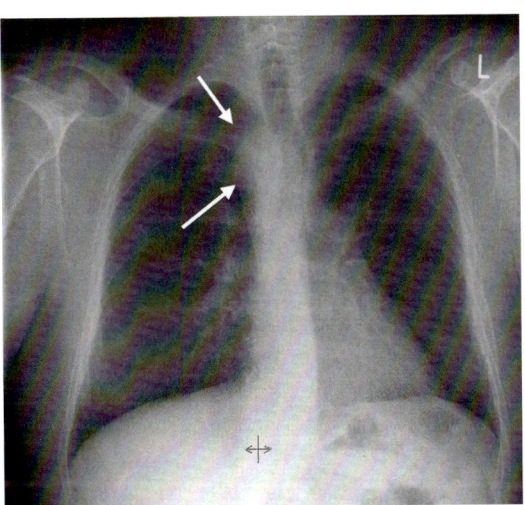

Fig. 9.15 Right-sided aortic arch (arrow) in a 36-year-old man. Chest radiograph shows displacement of the trachea toward the left side.

▶ **What does the clinician want to know?**

Accompanying cardiac anomalies • Narrowing or displacement of the trachea, bronchus, or esophagus.

Differential Diagnosis

Looping of the left pulmonary artery (pulmonary sling)	– Compression of the posterior trachea and anterior circumference of the esophagus
Vena cava compression syndrome	– Anterior tracheal compression – No esophageal compression

Tips and Pitfalls

A right-sided descending aortic arch is not necessarily associated with a serious congenital defect.

Selected References

Borth-Bruns T, Eichler A (eds.). Pädiatrische Kardiologie. Berlin, Heidelberg: Springer; 2004

Davies M, Guest PJ. Developmental abnormalities of the great vessels of the thorax and their embryological basis. Br J Radiol 2003; 76: 491–502

Hernanz-Schulman M. Vascular rings: a practical approach to imaging diagnosis. Pediatr Radiol 2005; 35: 961–979

Ito H et al. Double aortic arch with atresia, tapering and aneurysm of the left arch. Br J Radiol 2006; 79:e71–4

Oddone M et al. Multi-modality evaluation of the abnormalities of the aortic arches in children: techniques and imaging spectrum with emphasis on MRI. Pediatr Radiol 2005; 35: 947–960

Russo V et al. Congenital diseases of the thoracic aorta. Role of MRI and MRA. Eur Radiol 2006; 16: 676–684

Definition

▶ **Epidemiology**
Accounts for 1–3 % of all congenital cardiac anomalies.
▶ **Pathophysiology**
Depends on the underlying anomaly.
▶ **Pathoanatomy**
Two subtypes are distinguished:
- *Asplenia syndrome:* Asplenia • Ipsilateral inferior vena cava and aorta • Bilateral superior venae cavae • Three lobes in each lung • Anomalous pulmonary venous drainage • Severe cyanotic heart defect (AVSD, DORV, TGA, pulmonary stenosis, or atresia).
- *Polysplenia syndrome:* Polysplenia • Dilated azygos vein • No infrahepatic inferior vena cava • Bilateral superior venae cavae • Two lobes in each lung • Less severe cardiac malformation (common atrium, VSD).

Imaging Signs

▶ **Modality of choice**
Echocardiography for diagnosing the cardiac anomaly • MRI in older patients.
▶ **Chest radiograph and CT findings**
- *Asplenia syndrome:* Small interlobar fissure on each side • Cardiomegaly • Pulmonary edema.
- *Polysplenia syndrome:* No small interlobar fissure • Broad carinal angle • Prominent azygos vein • Inferior vena cava not visible in the lateral projection.
▶ **Echocardiographic and MRI findings**
Segmental description of cardiac anatomy in the context of the underlying anomaly • Anomalous pulmonary venous drainage • Ventricular function • Pressures in the pulmonary circulation can be assessed by color Doppler • *MRI:* Quantification of flow (phase-contrast imaging) to determine possible shunt volumes.
▶ **Invasive diagnostic procedures**
Indication depends on the underlying complex cardiac anomaly • Angiography may be done to visualize and quantify shunt flow • Systematic invasive pressure measurements may be taken preoperatively in the cardiac chambers and great vessels.

Clinical Aspects

▶ **Typical presentation**
Asplenia syndrome: Severe cyanosis • Pulmonary infections • Possible malrotation with volvulus, absent gallbladder, and extrahepatic biliary atresia.

▶ **Treatment options**
- *Asplenia syndrome:* Prostaglandin E_1 to maintain patency of a patent ductus arteriosus • Antibiotics • Early surgical biventricular correction is desired • Univentricular correction (Fontan procedure) may be appropriate.
- *Polysplenia syndrome:* Anastomosis of the azygos vein to the pulmonary circulation.

▶ **Course and prognosis**
Mortality in untreated newborns is 85% in asplenia syndrome and 65% in polysplenia syndrome during the first year of life.

▶ **What does the clinician want to know?**
Right isomerism (three lobes in each lung, asplenia, liver in the midline) • Left isomerism (two lobes in each lung, polysplenia, liver in the midline) • Anatomy • Functional and hemodynamic status of the associated, often complex cardiac anomaly.

Differential Diagnosis

Complete transposition of the viscera	– Mirror-image arrangement of all organs
	– Usually no cardiac anomalies
	– Associated with Kartagener syndrome
Dextroversion of the heart	– Heart on the right side of the chest
	– Cardiac apex still points toward the left

Tips and Pitfalls

Complex anomalies including congenital heart defects are commonly detected in utero by prenatal ultrasound. A congenital heart defect should always be considered in clinically abnormal infants and excluded by early echocardiography.

Selected References

Applegate KE et al. Situs revisited: imaging of the heterotaxy syndrome. Radiographics 1999; 19: 837–852; discussion 853–854

Borth-Bruns T, Eichler A (eds.). Pädiatrische Kardiologie. Berlin, Heidelberg: Springer; 2004

Winer-Muram HT. Adult presentation of heterotaxic syndromes and related complexes. J Thorac Imaging 1995; 10: 43–57

Winer-Muram HT, Tonkin IL. The spectrum of heterotaxic syndromes. Radiol Clin North Am 1989; 27: 1147–1170

Definition

▶ **Epidemiology**
Accounts for 3% of all congenital cardiac anomalies • 30% of patients have associated anomalies (coarctation of the aorta, persistent left superior vena cava).

▶ **Pathoanatomy**
Tricuspid valve is absent or membranous • Interatrial connection is necessary for life • PFO is usually present • Great vessels arise in a normal or transposed position • Development of the RV and pulmonary trunk depends on the presence and size of a VSD.

▶ **Pathophysiology**
A left-to-right shunt at the atrial and ventricular level (through a VSD) leads to ductal-independent perfusion of the lungs • Lung perfusion otherwise occurs through a PDA • Cyanosis is present due to blood mixing in the LA.

Imaging Signs

▶ **Modality of choice**
Echocardiography • MRI in older patients (postoperative follow-up).

▶ **Chest radiograph findings**
Cardiomegaly • Variable pulmonary vascular markings.

▶ **Echocardiographic and MRI findings**
Atrial size • Determination of pressure gradient across the VSD (color Doppler) • LV function.

▶ **Invasive diagnostic procedures**
Pulmonary angiography and invasive pressure measurement are indicated in rare cases.

Clinical Aspects

▶ **Typical presentation**
The dominant clinical feature may be cyanosis or heart failure, depending on the degree of lung perfusion • Critical condition results from ductal dependence and constriction of the PDA • Hypoxemic episodes in older children • Sequelae of chronic cyanosis and polyglobulia (stroke, brain abscess, coagulation disorders).

▶ **Treatment options**
Possible indication for prostaglandin E_1 • Treatment for heart failure • Endocarditis prophylaxis • The Rashkind procedure may be indicated in patients with a small interatrial connection with high pressure gradient • Fontan procedure for palliative surgical treatment.

▶ **Course and prognosis**
Untreated, 80–90% of affected infants will die before 1 year of age • Long-term Fontan-specific problems result from surgical palliation.

▶ **What does the clinician want to know?**
Position of the great arteries • Size of the cardiac chambers • ASD • VSD • LV function • Signs of pulmonary hypertension • Mitral valve function.

Fig. 9.16 Diagrammatic illustration of tricuspid atresia. A connection is established between the atria and ventricles, allowing the mixing of oxygenated and deoxygenated blood. The RV is hypoplastic.

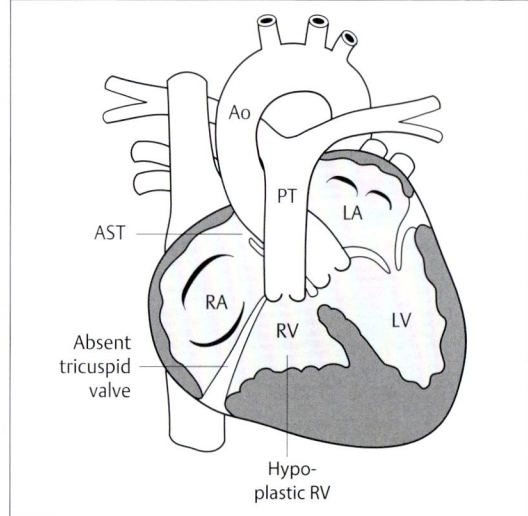

Fig. 9.17 Tricuspid atresia. SSFP image in the four-chamber view shows absence of the tricuspid valve (long arrow) and a hypoplastic RV (arrow) with an ASD between the RA and dilated LA (arrowhead).

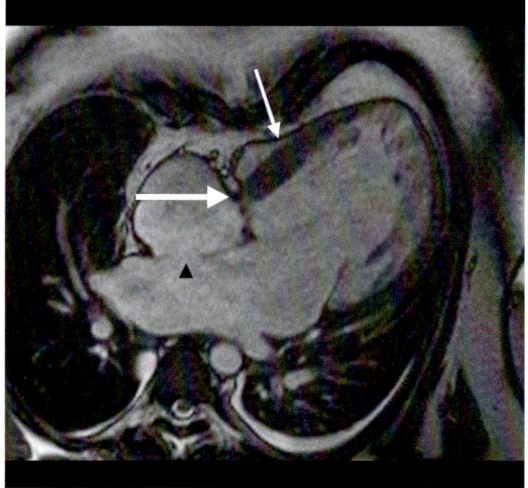

Differential Diagnosis

Ebstein anomaly	– Tricuspid valve displaced toward the cardiac apex
	– Large RA
	– RV is small but present

Selected References

Borth-Bruns T, Eichler A (eds.). Pädiatrische Kardiologie. Berlin, Heidelberg: Springer; 2004

Freedom RM et al. The Fontan procedure: analysis of cohorts and late complications. Cardiol Young 2000; 10: 307–331

Martinez RM, Anderson RH. Echo-morphological correlates in atrioventricular valvar atresia. Cardiol Young 2006; 16 Suppl 1: 27–34

Warnes CA. Tricuspid atresia and univentricular heart after the Fontan procedure. Cardiol Clin 1993; 11: 665–673

Definition

▶ **Epidemiology**
Accounts for less than 1% of all congenital cardiac anomalies • Commonly associated with a right descending aortic arch (30–40%) and DiGeorge syndrome.

▶ **Pathoanatomy**
The coronary, systemic, and pulmonary vasculature arise from a common arterial trunk • Large perimembranous VSD is located directly below the origin of the truncus • Bicuspid, tricuspid, or quadricuspid truncal valve • Frequent valvular insufficiency • Often combined with coronary and aortic arch anomalies.

Imaging Signs

▶ **Modality of choice**
Echocardiography.

▶ **Chest radiograph findings**
Cardiomegaly • Prominent pulmonary vasculature • Narrow mediastinum • A right descending aortic arch may be seen.

▶ **Echocardiographic findings**
Echocardiography can demonstrate the truncus arteriosus arising from both ventricles • High VSD • Common truncal valve • Ventricular and valvular function can be studied and quantified.

▶ **CT findings**
CTA can show the pulmonary arteries arising from the common trunk and can define their relationship to the MAPCA.

▶ **MRI findings**
Same as echocardiographic findings • Can accurately define the morphology of the thoracic vessels including the pulmonary arteries and MAPCA (MRA) • Quantification of valvular insufficiency (phase-contrast imaging).

▶ **Invasive diagnostic procedures**
Rarely necessary in the initial workup • Simultaneous opacification of the aorta and pulmonary arteries • Invasive contrast studies can exclude coronary abnormalities • Invasive pressure measurement may be indicated.

Clinical Aspects

▶ **Typical presentation**
Symptoms of heart failure are noted during the first days and weeks of life, caused predominantly by a large left-to-right shunt • Almost all children with truncus arteriosus will die in 6–12 months without operative treatment.

▶ **Treatment options**
Primary corrective surgery during the first days of life • The RV is connected to the pulmonary trunk or pulmonary arteries via a conduit or allograft (Rastelli operation) • Closure of the VSD with a patch • Reconstruction of the aortic arch • Low mortality in uncomplicated corrections (approximately 5–10%).

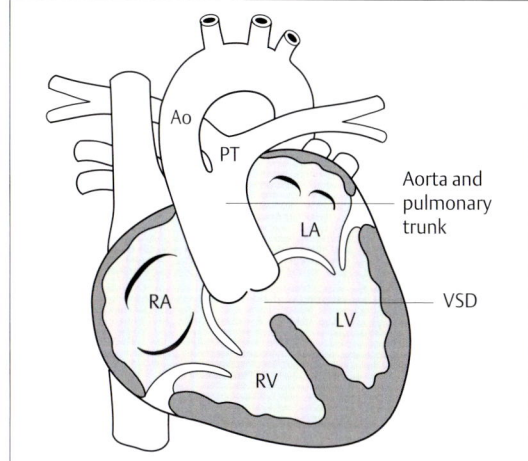

Fig. 9.18 Diagrammatic illustration of a truncus arteriosus (type I) with a common truncal valve overriding a high VSD. The aorta and pulmonary trunk (which divides into the left and right pulmonary arteries) both arise from the common arterial trunk. The mixing of blood in the ventricles and common trunk leads to cyanosis.

▶ **Course and prognosis**
One-year survival rate without operative treatment is approximately 10% • Clinical improvement is seen with (irreversible) recovery of pulmonary vascular resistance (at 3–4 months) • 10-year survival rate after corrective surgery is approximately 80%.

▶ **What does the clinician want to know?**
Estimated surgical risk • Truncal valve insufficiency • Coronary arterial anatomy • Possible pressure gradient across the stenotic pulmonary valve • MAPCA.

Differential Diagnosis

Aortopulmonary window	– Communication between the aorta and pulmonary artery due to a malformed aortopulmonary septum – Pulmonary valve and pulmonary artery are still present
TGA	– Pronounced cyanosis – Ductal-dependent – Earlier onset of symptoms

Selected References

Dorfman AL, Geva T. Magnetic resonance imaging evaluation of congenital heart disease: conotruncal anomalies. J Cardiovasc Magn Reson 2006; 8: 645–659

Momma K et al. Aortic arch anomalies associated with chromosome 22q11 deletion (CATCH 22). Pediatr Cardiol 1999; 20: 97–102

Rodefeld MD, Hanley FL. Neonatal truncus arteriosus repair: surgical techniques and clinical management. Semin Thorac Cardiovasc Surg Pediatr Card Surg Annu 2002; 5: 212–217

Tlaskal T et al. Repair of persistent truncus arteriosus with interrupted aortic arch. Eur J Cardiothorac Surg 2005; 28: 736–741

Definition

▶ **Epidemiology**
Very rare congenital cardiac anomaly (approximately 0.1%).

▶ **Etiology, pathophysiology, pathogenesis**
Incomplete incorporation of the embryonic common pulmonary vein into the wall of the left atrium • Corresponds functionally to mitral stenosis • Often associated with anomalous pulmonary venous drainage (10%), PDA, VSD, Shone complex, or Ebstein anomaly • Increased pressure in the left atrium with post-capillary pulmonary hypertension • The size of the opening between the accessory chamber and left atrium is of critical importance • Decreased cardiac output • Pressure overload on the right ventricle.

Imaging Signs

▶ **Modality of choice**
Echocardiography.

▶ **Chest radiograph findings**
Cardiomegaly • Chronic pulmonary vascular congestion • Possible acute pulmonary edema • Pleural effusion.

▶ **Echocardiographic findings**
Anatomic visualization of the pulmonary venous confluence • Determination of the pressure gradient across the opening • Evaluation of cardiac function (especially RV function) • Myocardial hypertrophy.

▶ **MRI and CT findings**
Cardiac anatomy • Accessory atrial chamber • MRI is better for excluding other vascular and cardiac anomalies • Precise evaluation of RV and LV function • May detect accelerated flow through the anomalous opening (blood jet).

▶ **Invasive diagnostic procedures**
Invasive pressure measurement may be indicated in patients with suspected pulmonary hypertension.

Clinical Aspects

▶ **Typical presentation**
Early symptoms of pulmonary congestion • Right-sided heart failure • Cardiac arrhythmias • Recurrent lung infections • Tachypnea • Chronic cough.

▶ **Treatment options**
Medical stabilization of heart failure • Anticoagulation in patients with atrial fibrillation • The accessory chamber is surgically opened and broadly anastomosed to the posterior wall of the LA.

▶ **Course and prognosis**
A small proportion of patients who undergo corrective surgery will develop refractory pulmonary venous stenosis with a poor prognosis • 80–90% of patients have normal life expectancy.

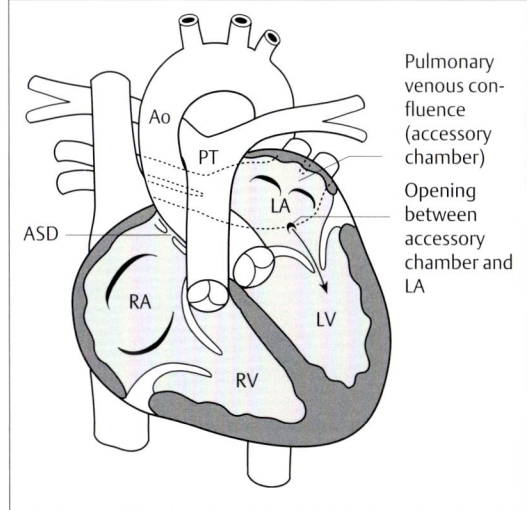

Pulmonary venous confluence (accessory chamber)

Opening between accessory chamber and LA

Fig. 9.19 Diagrammatic illustration of cor triatriatum. The pulmonary venous confluence forms an accessory chamber that communicates with the LA by a small opening that obstructs pulmonary venous flow (functional mitral stenosis).

▶ **What does the clinician want to know?**

Size of the opening ● Pulmonary hypertension ● Associated anomalies.

Differential Diagnosis

Valvular mitral stenosis   – Normal cardiac anatomy
                               – Morphologic changes in the mitral valve

Tips and Pitfalls

Some patients with a hemodynamically mild anomaly may reach adulthood before their condition is diagnosed (this is less common today owing to the widespread use of echocardiography).

Selected References

Borth-Bruns T, Eichler A (eds.). Pädiatrische Kardiologie. Berlin, Heidelberg: Springer; 2004

Goel AK et al. Atrioventricular septal defect with cor triatriatum: case report and review of the literature. Pediatr Cardiol 1998; 19: 243–245

Sakamoto I et al. Cine-magnetic resonance imaging of cor triatriatum. Chest 1994; 106: 1586–1589

Slight RD et al. Cor-triatriatum sinister presenting in the adult as mitral stenosis: an analysis of factors which may be relevant in late presentation. Heart Lung Circ 2005; 14: 8–12

Definition

▶ **Definition**
A very rare form of partial anomalous pulmonary venous drainage. All or part of the pulmonary vessels on the right side empty into a vein that drains into the inferior vena cava at the level of the diaphragm. The collecting vessel produces a convex shadow on the radiograph, resembling a curved Turkish sword (scimitar).

▶ **Epidemiology**
A quarter of patients have associated anomalies ● ASD (common) ● VSD ● TOF ● PDA ● Possible malformations of the diaphragm.

▶ **Etiology, pathophysiology, pathogenesis**
Left-to-right shunt to the RA (corresponds to the pathophysiology of ASD).

▶ **Pathoanatomy**
Hypoplasia of the right lung ● Anomalous communication of the right pulmonary veins with the inferior vena cava (partial anomalous pulmonary venous drainage).

Imaging Signs

▶ **Modality of choice**
Chest radiograph (spot diagnosis).

▶ **Chest radiograph and CT findings**
Hypoplasia of the right lung ● Possible dextroversion of the heart (not dextrocardia) ● Prominent RA ● Scimitar vein ● CT is useful for further investigation of pulmonary status.

▶ **Echocardiographic findings**
Termination of the scimitar vein ● No right pulmonary veins draining into the LA ● Exclusion of other cardiac anomalies.

▶ **MRI findings**
Same as echocardiographic findings ● Visualization of the scimitar vein ● Quantification of the shunt volume ● Contrast-enhanced MRA can provide a general survey view.

▶ **Invasive diagnostic procedures**
May demonstrate an atypical arterial supply to the right lung (from the celiac trunk, right renal artery, or descending aorta) ● Scimitar vein opacifies during the venous phase of pulmonary angiography.

Clinical Aspects

▶ **Typical presentation**
Symptoms are age-dependent:
– *Newborns:* Heart failure ● Right heart volume overload ● Pulmonary hypertension.
– *Children:* Frequent pulmonary infections ● Symptoms depend on the size of the shunt.

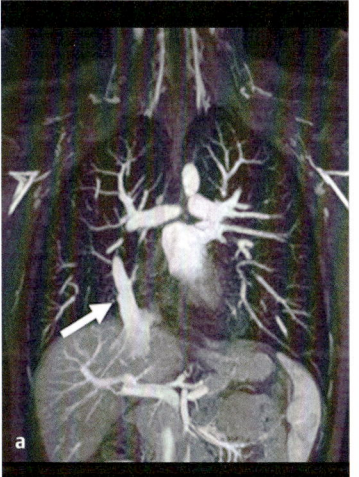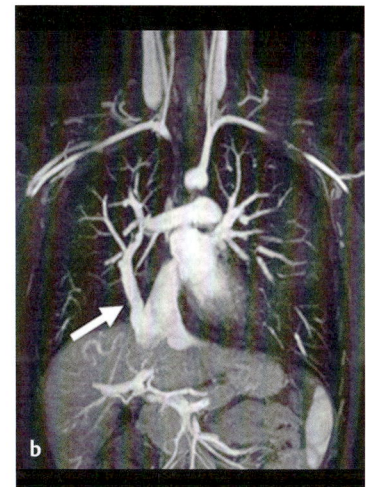

Fig. 9.20 a, b Contrast-enhanced MR angiographic image of scimitar syndrome. Coronal images (thin-slab MIP, **b**) show the scimitar vein draining into the inferior vena cava (arrow) (with kind permission of J. P. Finn, Los Angeles).

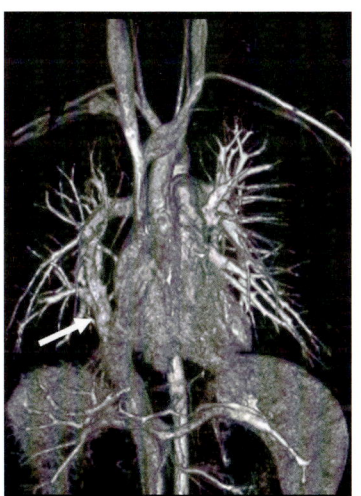

Fig. 9.21 Contrast-enhanced MR angiographic image (VRT) in the same patient as in Fig. 9.**20** demonstrates the connection of the scimitar vein to the inferior vena cava (arrow) (with kind permission of J. P. Finn, Los Angeles).

Fig. 9.22 Scimitar syndrome and dextrocardia. P-A chest radiograph shows absence of the cardiac silhouette on the left side. The scimitar vein can be identified on the right side, draining into the inferior vena cava (arrows).

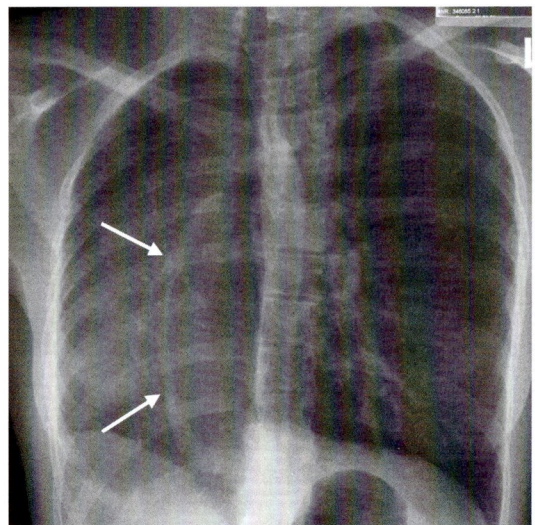

▶ **Treatment options**
Treatment depends on the shunt volume ● Anastomosis of the right pulmonary vein(s) to the left atrium ● Interventional embolization of atypical arterial vessels supplying the right lung.

▶ **Course and prognosis**
Prognosis is fair to poor in symptomatic newborns ● Prognosis is good following corrective surgery and in asymptomatic adults.

▶ **What does the clinician want to know?**
Anatomic findings ● Shunt volumes ● Associated anomalies.

Differential Diagnosis

Other forms of partial anomalous pulmonary venous drainage	– Investigate pulmonary venous anatomy
Isolated hypoplasia of the right lung	– Normal termination of the pulmonary veins

Tips and Pitfalls

When scimitar syndrome is diagnosed incidentally (by chest radiograph) in patients with mild symptoms, further tests should be done to determine the hemodynamic significance of the anomaly.

Selected References

Kramer U et al. Scimitar syndrome: morphological diagnosis and assessment of hemodynamic significance by magnetic resonance imaging. Eur Radiol 2003; 13 [Suppl 4]: L147–150

Definition

▶ **Epidemiology**
Two percent of all congenital cardiac anomalies • Associated with trisomy 21 in 30–40% of cases • Most common associated anomalies are PDA (10%) and tetralogy of Fallot (approximately 6%).

▶ **Pathoanatomy and classification**
Partial AVSD: ASD I (ostium primum defect) • Intact ventricular septum • Cleft in the mitral valve • Two separate AV valve rings.
Complete AVSD: Usually features a common AV valve and large VSD • 50% of cases have mitral insufficiency • Possible ventricular hypoplasia.

▶ **Etiology, pathophysiology, pathogenesis**
RV pressures are only moderately elevated in partial AVSD • Complete AVSD is often associated with a large left-to-right shunt that equalizes the pressures between the RV and LV.

Imaging Signs

▶ **Modality of choice**
Echocardiography.

▶ **Chest radiograph findings**
Cardiomegaly • Prominent pulmonary segment • Increased pulmonary vascular markings • Increased interstitial markings in patients with heart failure.

▶ **Echocardiographic findings**
Size and location of the ASD and VSD • Anatomy of the valves • AV valve opening • Size and function of the RV and LV.

▶ **MRI findings**
Cardiac anatomy • Cardiac function • Estimation of the shunt volume by flowmetry in the pulmonary artery and ascending aorta • Detection of concomitant valvular insufficiency.

▶ **Invasive diagnostic procedures**
Rarely necessary during the initial workup • Invasive pressure measurement is indicated in patients with suspected pulmonary hypertension.

Clinical Aspects

▶ **Typical presentation**
Patients with a small partial AVSD are often asymptomatic • A complete AVSD in infants leads to heart failure • Atrial arrhythmias • Manifestations of AV block • Pulmonary infections • Subaortic stenosis • Prolonged AV conduction • RV hypertrophy • Occasional complete RBBB.

▶ **Treatment options**
Medical treatment for overt heart failure • Endocarditis prophylaxis in exposed patients • Surgical closure in patients with persistent atrial arrhythmias, impaired ventricular function, an incompetent left AV valve, or significant subaortic stenosis • Surgical closure of a complete AVSD should be done during the first year of life • Reconstruction of the AV valves.

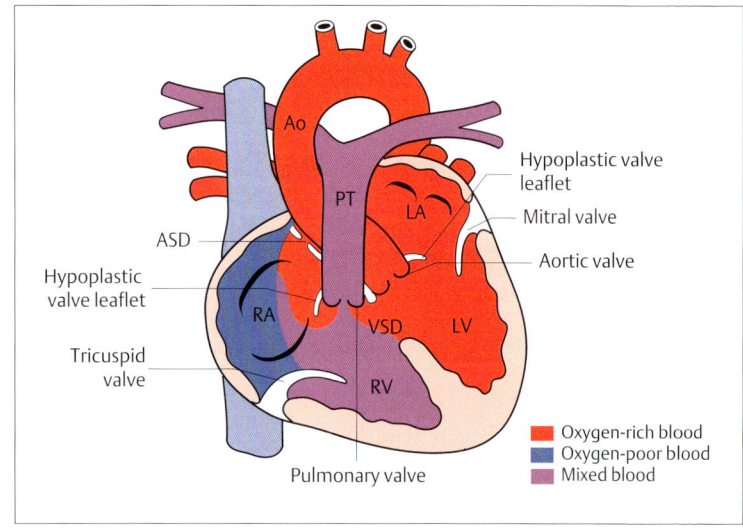

Fig. 9.23 Diagrammatic illustration of a complete AVSD with an ASD (ostium primum) and a high perimembranous VSD.

Fig. 9.24 Echocardiogram of AVSD. Four-chamber view shows a complete defect of the septum primum (arrow) and perimembranous septum (arrowheads) (with kind permission of L. Sieverding, Tübingen).

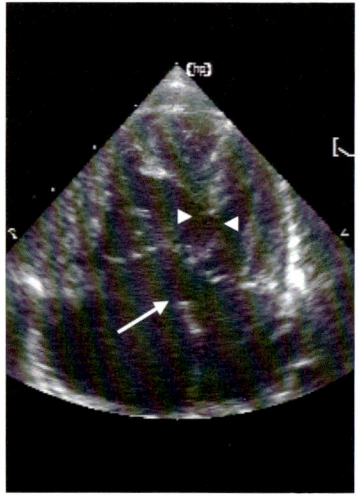

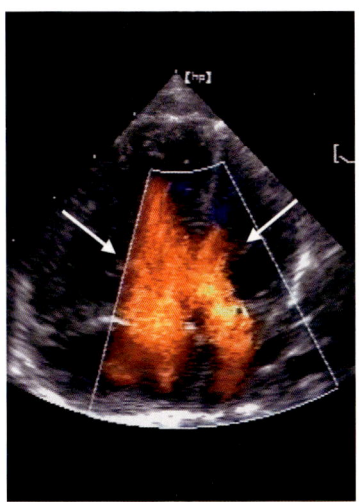

Fig. 9.25 Color Doppler image from the same patient as in Fig. 9.**24**. Four-chamber view demonstrates a systolic shunt between the left and right ventricles (arrow) (with kind permission of L. Sieverding, Tübingen).

▶ **Course and prognosis**
A complete AVSD causes irreversible pulmonary hypertension by 6–12 months of age ● Perioperative mortality is 5–10% ● *Postoperative complications:* Mitral insufficiency or stenosis (5–10%), subaortic stenosis (< 5%), complete AV block, and sinus node dysfunction.

▶ **What does the clinician want to know?**
Morphological status ● Partial or complete AVSD ● Valvular and ventricular function ● Shunt volume ● Signs of heart failure.

Differential Diagnosis

Isolated ASD or VSD (may have similar clinical manifestations, depending on the shunt volume).

Selected References

Borth-Bruns T, Eichler A (eds.). Pädiatrische Kardiologie. Berlin, Heidelberg: Springer; 2004

Brickner ME, Hillis LD, Lange RA. Congenital heart disease in adults: first of two parts. N Engl J Med 2000; 342: 256–263

Craig B. Atrioventricular septal defect: from fetus to adult. Heart 2006; 92: 1879–1885

McCarthy KP et al. Perimembranous and muscular ventricular septal defects—morphology revisited in the era of device closure. J Interv Cardiol 2005; 18: 507–513

Meisner H, Guenther T. Atrioventricular septal defect. Pediatr Cardiol 1998; 19: 276–281

Quaegebeur JM, Cooper RS. Surgery for atrioventricular septal defects. Adv Cardiol 2004; 41: 127–132

Wang ZJ et al. Cardiovascular shunts: MR imaging evaluation. Radiographics 2003; 23 Spec No: S181–S194

Definition

▶ **Epidemiology**

Rare congenital cardiac anomaly (< 1%) • Males and females are affected equally.

▶ **Pathoanatomy**

Anatomic and functional defects of the tricuspid valve • Tricuspid valve is displaced into the RV, leading to tricuspid insufficiency • The RV and RVOT are enlarged • Shunt at the atrial level (PFO or ASD II) is present in 50% • Accessory conduction pathways with risk of AV reentry tachycardia in 25% of cases • *Common associated anomalies:* VSD, pulmonary stenosis, mitral valve prolapse, coarctation of the aorta.

▶ **Etiology, pathophysiology, pathogenesis**

RV hypoplasia with fibrosis, dilatation, and secondary heart failure • Dilatation of the RA, predisposing to arrhythmias.

Imaging Signs

▶ **Modality of choice**

Echocardiography • MRI in older patients.

▶ **Chest radiograph findings**

Advanced dilatation of the RA ("globular-shaped heart") • Small vascular segment • Cardiac configuration similar to that in pericardial effusion.

▶ **Echocardiographic findings**

Apical displacement of the tricuspid valve by more than 8 mm/m^2 body surface area • Elongated, "flailing" anterior valve leaflet • Large RA with a small, atrialized RV • Tricuspid insufficiency.

▶ **MRI findings**

Same as echocardiographic findings • Useful in older patients, as it can often define the RV more clearly than echocardiograms.

▶ **Invasive diagnostic procedures**

Rarely necessary in the initial workup.

Clinical Aspects

▶ **Typical presentation**

Affected newborns often have cyanosis and heart failure due to the right-to-left shunt • Older patients exhibit clubbing of the fingers • Dyspnea • Fatigue • Supraventricular arrhythmias • Syncopal attacks • Hepatomegaly • Impulse conduction disorders with a complete RBBB and a right anterior hemiblock • First-degree AV block (in up to 40% of patients) • WPW syndrome (in up to 20% of patients).

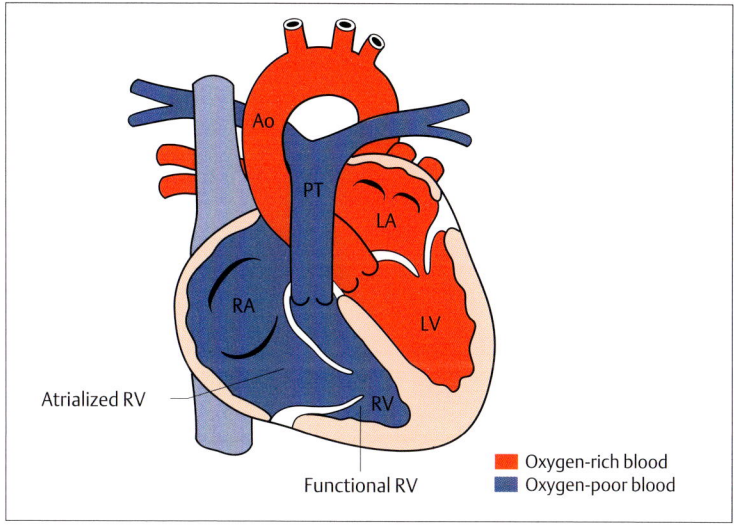

Fig. 9.26 Diagrammatic illustration of Ebstein anomaly. The posterior leaflet of the tricuspid valve is displaced into the RV. The free wall of the RV is thin and dilated, and the right ventricular inflow tract is incorporated into the RA ("atrialized").

▶ **Treatment options**
Cyanotic newborns may require prostaglandin E_1 therapy to maintain ductal patency • Medical management of heart failure • Endocarditis prophylaxis • Acute adenosine for AV reentry tachycardia • Prophylaxis with β-blockers or verapamil • WPW syndrome may require catheter ablation, tricuspid valvuloplasty, or tricuspid valve replacement in patients with progressive cardiomegaly, cyanosis, TIA, stroke, or severe tricuspid insufficiency • ASD repair is an option in patients with extreme RV hypoplasia; Fontan procedure or bidirectional cavopulmonary (Glenn) anastomosis is available for palliation • High surgical risk • Some patients may require heart transplantation.
Aftercare: Endocarditis prophylaxis • Avoidance of sports activities • Follow-ups at short intervals, giving particular attention to arrhythmias.

▶ **Course and prognosis**
Predictors of increased mortality include NYHA class, cardiac size, cyanosis, and paroxysmal atrial tachycardia.

▶ **What does the clinician want to know?**
Precise morphological description • Functional status of the tricuspid valve (incompetent?) • Right-to-left shunt through an ASD.

Differential Diagnosis

Large ASD	– No cyanosis
	– Increased pulmonary blood flow
	– Left-to-right shunt
Pericardial effusion	– No cyanosis
	– Easily distinguished by echocardiography

Tips and Pitfalls

The follow-up of RV and LV hemodynamic functional parameters is important in assessing response to treatment ● NYHA class is a useful prognostic factor.

Selected References

Brickner ME, Hillis LD, Lange RA. Congenital heart disease in adults: second of two parts. N Engl J Med 2000; 342(5): 334–342

Definition

▶ **Epidemiology**

Six percent of congenital cardiac anomalies • Most common cyanotic heart defect in children • Frequently associated with DiGeorge syndrome (microdeletion 22q11).

▶ **Pathoanatomy, pathophysiology**

Cyanotic heart defect involving a combination of severe pulmonary stenosis, RV hypertrophy, a subaortic VSD, and a dilated aorta that overrides the interventricular septum • Many patients have associated anomalies • Right aortic arch (25%) • Coronary anomalies (5–10%, may require attention during corrective heart surgery) • ASD (10%).

▶ **Etiology, pathophysiology, pathogenesis**

A large VSD equalizes the pressures between the ventricles • Some venous blood does not enter the lungs but reenters the systemic circulation in a deoxygenated state (cyanosis) • Hemodynamics and symptoms are determined by the right-to-left shunt, the severity of the RVOT obstruction, and associated anomalies • A rise in systemic vascular resistance reduces the right-to-left shunt, decreasing the severity of cyanosis.

Imaging Signs

▶ **Modality of choice**

Echocardiography • MRI is useful in older patients and for pre- and postoperative evaluation.

▶ **Chest radiograph findings**

"Boot-shaped" heart • RV hypertrophy • Decreased pulmonary vascular markings • Possible right aortic arch (25%).

▶ **Echocardiographic findings**

Visualization of the VSD • Position of the aortic root and aortic arch • Function of the pulmonary valve • RVOT obstruction • Pulmonary vascular anatomy • Other associated anomalies.

▶ **CT and MRI findings**

Postoperative morphologic evaluation • Detection of MAPCA • MRI is comparable with echocardiography, especially in terms of functional findings • Visualization of postoperative status (e.g., after a Blalock–Taussig shunt) • Assessment of shunt patency • MRI is usually better than echocardiography for determining flow volume and regurgitant fraction (MRA, flow quantification by phase-contrast imaging) • Precise evaluation of RV function and myocardial hypertrophy.

▶ **Invasive diagnostic procedures**

May be used to define coronary anatomy • Quantification of the VSD • Intervention for pulmonary stenosis • Preoperative embolization of MAPCA.

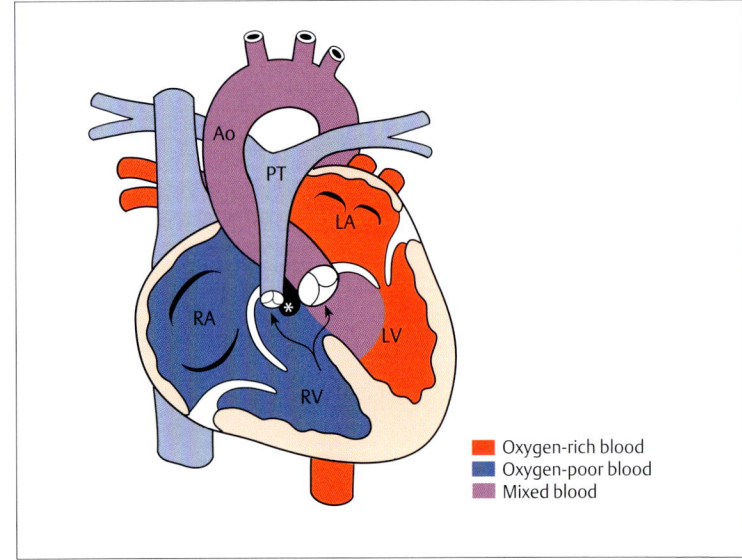

Fig. 9.27 Diagrammatic illustration of tetralogy of Fallot—subvalvular pulmonary stenosis (muscle, *) with a small pulmonary valve, a large aortic valve overriding a high VSD, and right ventricular hypertrophy. The right-to-left shunt leads to cyanosis.

Oxygen-rich blood
Oxygen-poor blood
Mixed blood

Clinical Aspects

▶ **Typical presentation**
Children: Cyanosis • Possible hypoxemic episodes • Typical squatting position in older children (increases systemic vascular resistance) • Polyglobulia • Clubbing of the fingers • Hour-glass deformity of the nails.
Adults: Dyspnea • Decreased exercise tolerance • Chronic cyanosis • Brain abscess • Stroke • Endocarditis.

▶ **Treatment options**
Hypoxemic episodes can be interrupted by physical measures and heavy sedation • β-blockers for prophylaxis • Digitalization is contraindicated • Without surgical intervention, most patients die in childhood • Corrective surgery should be done as soon as possible to prevent secondary damage to the heart, lungs, and CNS • Surgery may be done in infancy (patch repair of VSD, expansion of the RVOT, commissurotomy, transannular patch repair, mortality < 5%) • In severe hypoplasia of the pulmonary arteries, a palliative shunt can be placed between the subclavian artery and pulmonary artery (modified Blalock–Taussig shunt) • Interventional balloon valvuloplasty and stent implantation are accepted as standard treatments.

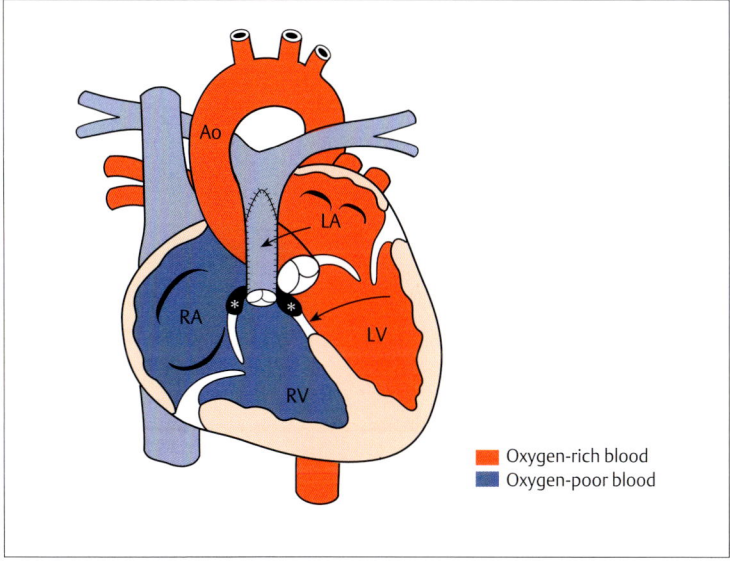

Fig. 9.28   Diagrammatic illustration of surgically corrected TOF. The VSD is repaired with a patch (long arrow). The opening between the RV and PT is enlarged by surgical removal of the subvalvular stenosis (muscle *) and hypoplastic pulmonary artery and by reconstruction of the PT (short arrow). If a palliative Blalock–Taussig shunt was placed in a previous operation, it is removed in the second operation.

▶ **Course and prognosis**

Corrective surgery is still advised in patients who have reached adulthood without operative treatment ● Patients with corrected TOF are usually asymptomatic (approximately 85% survival rate 35 years after surgery).

Postoperative complications: Endocarditis ● Ventricular arrhythmias ● 15% of patients require a second operation, e.g., for a residual VSD with Q_p:Q_s > 1.5:1, severe pulmonary stenosis, pulmonary or aortic insufficiency, or an aneurysm of the RVOT or ascending aorta (> 55 mm).

Aftercare: Endocarditis prophylaxis ● Surveillance of valvular function ● Surveillance of a residual VSD ● Observation for cardiac arrhythmias.

▶ **What does the clinician want to know?**

Degree of RVOT obstruction ● Anatomy of the RVOT ● Magnitude of the right-to-left shunt ● Origin and course of the coronary arteries ● Development of pulmonary vessels (important for surgical planning).

Fig. 9.29 MR image in a patient with tetralogy of Fallot. Cine GRE sequence demonstrates RV hypertrophy (arrowheads), a ventricular septal defect (short arrow), and an overriding aorta (long arrow).

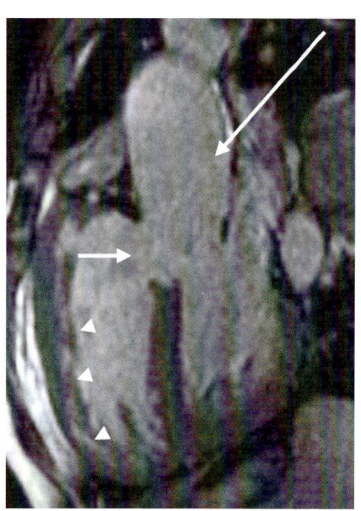

Differential Diagnosis

Other cardiac anomalies   – Pulmonary atresia
                                     – Truncus arteriosus
                                     – DORV

Selected References

Borth-Bruns T, Eichler A (eds.). Pädiatrische Kardiologie. Berlin, Heidelberg: Springer; 2004

Brickner ME, Hillis LD, Lange RA. Congenital heart disease in adults: second of two parts. N Engl J Med 2000; 342(5): 334–342

Dorfman AL, Geva T. Magnetic resonance imaging evaluation of congenital heart disease: conotruncal anomalies. J Cardiovasc Magn Reson 2006; 8: 645–659

Haramati LB et al. MR imaging and CT of vascular anomalies and connections in patients with congenital heart disease: significance in surgical planning. Radiographics 2002; 22: 337–47; discussion 348–349

Pokorski RJ. Long-term survival after repair of tetralogy of Fallot. J Insur Med 2000; 32: 89–92

Shinebourne EA et al. Tetralogy of Fallot: from fetus to adult. Heart 2006; 92: 1353–1359

Therrien J et al. Late problems in tetralogy of Fallot—recognition, management, and prevention. Cardiol Clin 2002; 20: 395–404

Williams RG et al; National Heart, Lung, and Blood Institute Working Group on research in adult congenital heart disease. Report of the National Heart, Lung, and Blood Institute Working Group on research in adult congenital heart disease. J Am Coll Cardiol 2006; 47: 701–707

Zannini L, Borini I. State of the art of cardiac surgery in patients with congenital heart disease. J Cardiovasc Med (Hagerstown) 2007; 8: 3–6

Definition

▶ **Epidemiology**

Seven to nine percent of all congenital cardiac anomalies • More common in males than in females (2:1) • Increased incidence in Turner syndrome.

▶ **Etiology, pathophysiology, pathogenesis**

Underdevelopment of the left heart • No impairment of fetal circulation • Severe obstruction of the LV and LVOT • Oxygenated blood from pulmonary veins enters the right atrium through the foramen ovale • Dilatation of the right heart and pulmonary arteries • Systemic perfusion occurs through the PDA.

Imaging Signs

▶ **Modality of choice**

Echocardiography • MRI and invasive studies for postoperative care (e.g., after the Fontan procedure).

▶ **Chest radiograph findings**

Cardiomegaly • Increased pulmonary venous markings • Possible congestion with interstitial edema • Narrow mediastinum.

▶ **Echocardiographic findings**

Decreased aortic diameter (< 5 mm) • Small LV • Dilatation of the right heart and pulmonary arteries • PDA • Duplex scan shows left-to-right shunt through the PFO • Echocardiography can be used to assess pressure relationships.

▶ **CT and MRI findings**

Used mainly for postoperative evaluations • Patency of aortopulmonary (Blalock–Taussig) shunt and cavopulmonary (Glenn) shunt • Pulmonary arterial anatomy • MR flowmetry for evaluation of cardiac and shunt function.

▶ **Invasive diagnostic procedures**

Can be used to detect coronary anomalies • Used mainly in postoperative follow-up • Flow visualization in the hypoplastic ascending aorta • Visualization of the connection of the pulmonary arteries through the PDA • Determination of postoperative pressure relationships.

Clinical Aspects

▶ **Typical presentation**

No clinical symptoms immediately after birth • Rapid deterioration after closure of the ductus arteriosus • Heart failure • Volume overload on the pulmonary circulation • Cardiogenic shock • Cyanosis.

▶ **Treatment options**

Prostaglandin E_1 to maintain ductal patency • With an interatrial defect small enough to maintain a pressure gradient, the ASD can be expanded by balloon dilatation (Rashkind atrioseptostomy) • Palliative surgical intervention by the Norwood procedure • Heart transplantation is advocated at some centers.

▶ **Course and prognosis**

Untreated newborns will die in a matter of days or weeks • Otherwise the prognosis depends on the course and complications of the Fontan procedure.

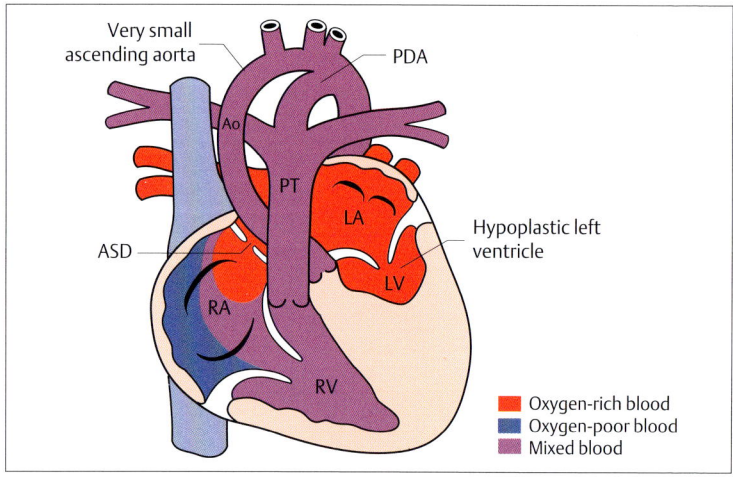

Fig. 9.30 Diagrammatic illustration of HLHS, characterized by hypoplasia of the LA, LV, aortic valve, and ascending aorta (type I). Blood is oxygenated by mixing in the RA with a left-to-right shunt through the ASD. Systemic blood flow relies on a PDA.

Fig. 9.31 MR image in a 6-month-old boy with HLHS. T1-weighted TSE sequence in an axial plane demonstrates a hypoplastic LV (arrow), an ASD (arrowheads), and a single, hypertrophic RV.

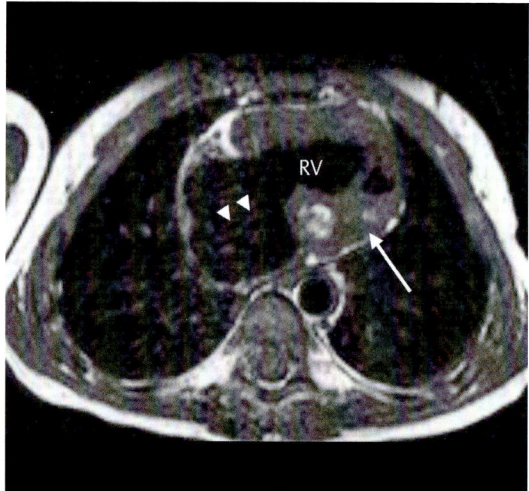

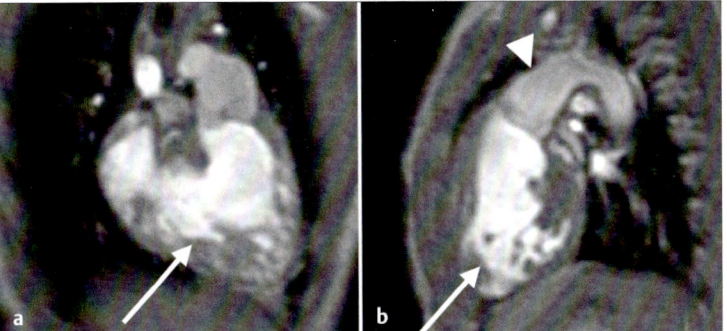

Fig. 9.32 a, b Same patient as in Fig. 9.**31**. Cine GRE sequence in an oblique coronal plane (**a**) and oblique sagittal plane (**b**). Note the hypertrophic single RV (arrow) and the functionally arterialized pulmonary artery (arrowhead) with a hypoplastic aorta. Blood is directed to the lungs through a Glenn or Fontan shunt (not shown).

▶ **What does the clinician want to know?**
Degree of LV and aortic hypoplasia • Size of the PDA and ASD • Ventricular function • Tricuspid insufficiency • Coronary anomalies.

Differential Diagnosis

Aortic stenosis, coarctation of the aorta, interrupted aortic arch	– LV pressure overload in a normally developed heart
Cardiomyopathy	– Generally enlarged heart with normal morphology – Myocardial dysfunction
Arteriovenous malformation	– Morphologically normal heart with volume overload of all chambers

Tips and Pitfalls

If a diagnosis is not made immediately after birth, HLHS should be suspected in infants who show progressive cyanosis and rapid clinical deterioration • Echocardiography should be scheduled as soon as possible.

Selected References

Alsoufi B et al. New developments in the treatment of hypoplastic left heart syndrome. Pediatrics 2007; 119: 109–117

Bardo DM et al. Hypoplastic left heart syndrome. Radiographics 2001; 21: 705–717

Bove EL et al. Hypoplastic left heart syndrome: conventional surgical management. Semin Thorac Cardiovasc Surg Pediatr Card Surg Annu 2004; 7: 3–10

Walker SG, Stuth EA. Single-ventricle physiology: perioperative implications. Semin Pediatr Surg 2004; 13: 188–202

Definition

▶ **Epidemiology**
Accounts for approximately 3% of all congenital cardiac anomalies.

▶ **Etiology, pathophysiology, pathogenesis**
Blood is delivered to the lungs through the ductus arteriosus and MAPCA • Cyanosis depends on blood mixing and the degree of pulmonary blood flow • Copious lung perfusion leads to heart failure.

▶ **Pathoanatomy**
Pulmonary atresia combined with a VSD and MAPCA • Some authors classify the condition as an extreme form of TOF • Persistence or hypertrophy of primitive arterial connections with the lung • Hypertrophy of the bronchial arteries.

Imaging Signs

▶ **Modality of choice**
Echocardiography • MRI in older patients.

▶ **Chest radiograph findings**
Conspicuous "boot-shaped" heart • Decreased pulmonary vascular markings • Small hila • Possible right descending aortic arch.

▶ **Echocardiographic findings**
Pulmonary atresia • Visualization of the pulmonary vessels • VSD • Overriding aortic root • Associated anomalies.

▶ **CT and MRI findings**
Most useful for demonstrating MAPCA and intracardiac anomalies • MRI and CT are excellent for defining the pulmonary arteries and for the postoperative exclusion of complications (stenosis of a shunt or conduit) • Phase-contrast MRI can be done if flowmetry is required.

▶ **Invasive diagnostic procedures**
Selective visualization of MAPCA • Invasive pressure measurement • Angiography may be done prior to interventional therapy (PTA of peripheral pulmonary artery stenosis, embolization of MAPCA) • Coronary angiography.

Clinical Aspects

▶ **Typical presentation**
Increasing cyanosis after closure of the ductus arteriosus • Heart failure due to large MAPCA • Clubbing of the fingers • Watchglass deformity of the nails • Dyspnea • Crouched or squatting position.

▶ **Treatment options**
Prostaglandin E_1 to maintain ductal patency • Palliative systemic–pulmonary arterial shunt (Blalock–Taussig) • Banding of MAPCA • Surgical creation of a conduit between the RV and pulmonary artery • Reconstruction of the RVOT • Repair of VSD (generally has a moderate to high surgical risk).

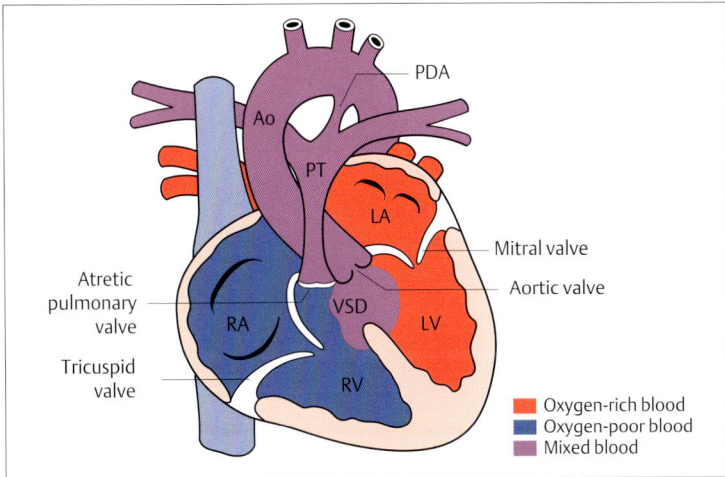

Fig. 9.33 Diagrammatic illustration of pulmonary atresia with an atretic pulmonary valve and blood mixing through a VSD (type I). The lungs receive mixed blood flow through a PDA.

▶ **Course and prognosis**
Life expectancy is less than 10 years without treatment ● Late problems are common after treatment ● Arrhythmias ● Conduit stenosis or leak ● Proximal stenosis of pulmonary arteries.

▶ **What does the clinician want to know?**
Location of the VSD ● Presence of PDA or collaterals ● Degree of pulmonary vascular hypoplasia ● AV valvular insufficiency ● Coronary anomaly.

Differential Diagnosis

TOF	– At least partial patency of the RVOT
Pulmonary atresia without a VSD	– Cyanosis
	– Tricuspid insufficiency
	– Massive dilatation of the RA
	– Small RV

Tips and Pitfalls

The pulmonary arterial supply and MAPCA are important prognostic indicators. They should be carefully assessed, therefore, if necessary by using a combination of modalities (MRI, CT).

Selected References

Amark KM et al. Independent factors associated with mortality, reintervention, and achievement of complete repair in children with pulmonary atresia with ventricular septal defect. J Am Coll Cardiol 2006; 47: 1448–1456

Bichell DP. Evaluation and management of pulmonary atresia with intact ventricular septum. Curr Opin Cardiol 1999; 14: 60–66

Boechat MI et al. Cardiac MR imaging and MR angiography for assessment of complex tetralogy of Fallot and pulmonary atresia. Radiographics 2005; 25: 1535–1546

Pourmoghadam KK et al. Congenital unilateral pulmonary venous atresia: definitive diagnosis and treatment. Pediatr Cardiol 2003; 24: 73–79

Definition

▶ **Epidemiology**
Four percent of all congenital cardiac anomalies ● Second most common cyanotic heart defect.

▶ **Pathoanatomy**
The great vessels arise from the "wrong" ventricles (ventriculoarterial discordance) ● Normal ventricular anatomy (atrioventricular concordance) ● Two forms are distinguished:
  – *Simple TGA* (approximately 2/3 of cases): Anomalous origin of the great arteries.
  – *Complex TGA:* Additional presence of a significant VSD ● Pulmonary stenosis ● Occasional coarctation of the aorta ● Coronary anomalies.

▶ **Etiology, pathophysiology, pathogenesis**
Parallel arrangement of both circulations ● Compatible with life only if defects (ASD, PDA, VSD) that are present allow the mixing of venous and arterial blood ● Postnatal ductal closure leads to early, severe hypoxemia.

Imaging Signs

▶ **Modality of choice**
Echocardiography ● MRI in older patients.

▶ **Chest radiograph findings**
Cardiomegaly ● Narrow mediastinum ● Prominent pulmonary vessels.

▶ **Echocardiographic findings**
Typical parallel arrangement of the great arteries in the parasternal short-axis view ● Visualization of cardiac anatomy (possible PFO, VSD, PDA).

▶ **CT findings**
Multidetector CT angiography can define ventriculoarterial anatomy ● Indicated mainly during the immediate postoperative period (if Echocardiographic findings are equivocal).

▶ **MRI findings**
3D MRA can define cardiac and ventriculoarterial anatomy in considerable detail ● May detect PFO, ASD, PDA, or pulmonary stenosis ● Postoperative follow-up after the Senning or Mustard procedure.

▶ **Invasive diagnostic procedures**
May be used to visualize the coronary arteries ● Invasive pressure measurement.

Clinical Aspects

▶ **Typical presentation**
Newborns present with cyanosis and severe heart failure.

▶ **Treatment options**
Newborns with hypoxemia due to a restrictive or closed PDA require immediate prostaglandin E_1 therapy ● Heart failure should be treated as required ● With an

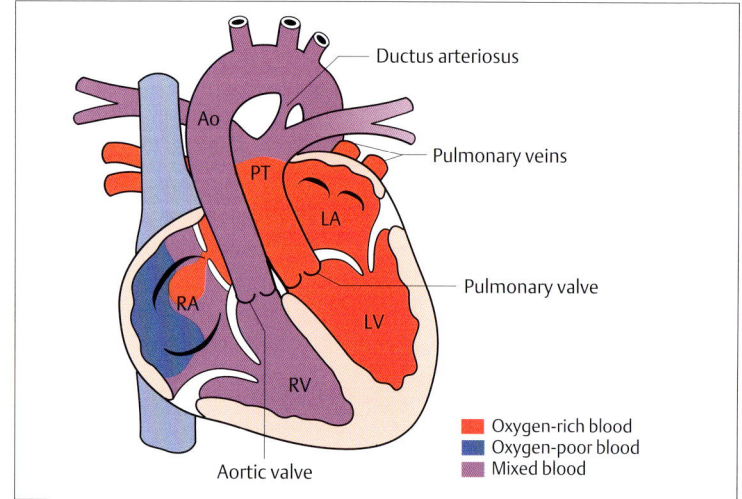

Fig. 9.34 Diagrammatic illustration of dextro-TGA, in which the aorta arises from the RV and the pulmonary artery arises from the LV. Mixing of blood occurs through an ASD and PDA.

interatrial defect small enough to maintain a pressure gradient, the ASD can be expanded by balloon dilatation (Rashkind atrioseptostomy).

Jatene arterial switch operation: Primary corrective procedure done during the first 2 weeks of life • Involves division of the great arteries, isolation of the coronary ostia, reanastomosis to the concordant ventricles, and reimplantation of the coronary arteries at the neoaortic root • The Lecompte maneuver (advancing the pulmonary bifurcation in front of the ascending aorta) is usually added • The surgical risk of an uncomplicated switch operation for TGA is less than 5% • The risk is markedly higher in complex forms.

Atrial switch operation of Senning or Mustard: Poorer long-term results • Should be considered only if the time window for an arterial switch has passed • Goal is to redirect pulmonary venous blood flow to the functional LV and systemic venous flow to the functional RV.

▶ **Course and prognosis**

One-year survival rate is less than 10% without operative treatment.

Arterial switch operation: Results in almost normal long-term survival. Postoperative complications: RVOT obstruction • Coronary stenosis • Arrhythmias • Ectasia of the neoaorta • Aortic or pulmonary valve insufficiency • Residual VSD.

Atrial switch: 25-year survival rate is approximately 80% in patients with a simple TGA.

Complications: Frequent arrhythmias • Stenosis of the atrium, vena cava, and pulmonary veins • Right ventricular dysfunction.

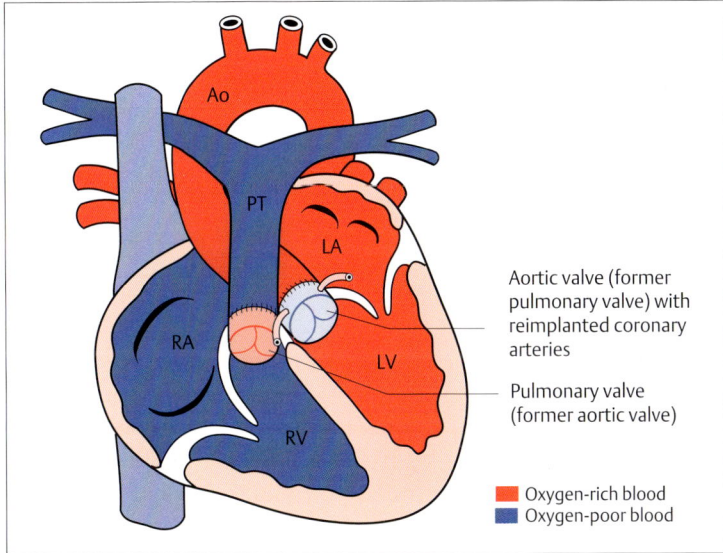

Fig. 9.35   Jatene arterial switch operation with reimplantation of the coronary arteries.

Aftercare: Endocarditis prophylaxis • Medical management of heart failure • Follow-up by ECG, echo, MRI, and cardiac catheterization.

▶ **What does the clinician want to know?**
Detailed description of anatomic relationships • Associated anomalies • Quantification of hemodynamic changes • Ventricular function.

Tips and Pitfalls
Regular follow-ups should be maintained after corrective surgery, including taking hemodynamic measurements, to determine the timing of any subsequent operation that may be needed.

Selected References
Brickner ME, Hillis LD, Lange RA. Congenital heart disease in adults: second of two parts. N Engl J Med 2000; 342(5): 334–342

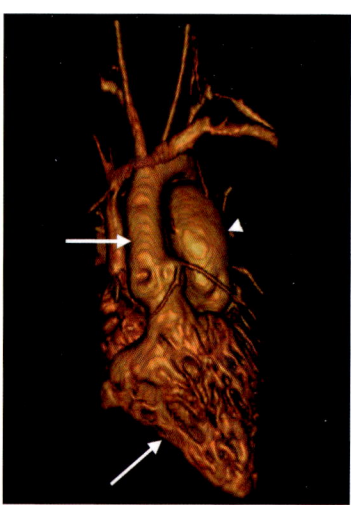

Fig. 9.36   Volume-rendered image from a 3D MRA study of dextro-TGA (anterior view) shows a trabecularized morphologic RV giving rise to the ascending aorta (arrow). The pulmonary artery arises from the morphologic LV (arrowhead).

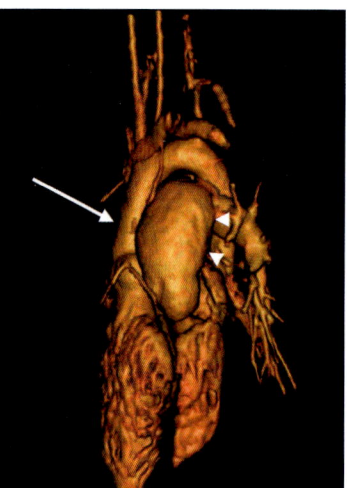

Fig. 9.37   Same patient as in Fig. 9.**36**. Left lateral view of the ascending aorta (arrow) and pulmonary artery (arrowhead).

Definition

▶ **Epidemiology**
Rare • Less than 4% of all congenital cardiac anomalies.

▶ **Etiology, pathophysiology, pathogenesis**
Pressure overload of the (anatomically right) systemic ventricle • Eventual failure • Atypical position of the AV node • Increased risk of AV block.

▶ **Pathoanatomy**
The cardiac chambers and great vessels are arranged in the following sequence: vena cava—right atrium—*left* ventricle—pulmonary arteries—pulmonary veins—left atrium—*right* ventricle—aorta • The aorta typically occupies an anomalous anterior position on the left side of the heart • Associated anomalies are common—malformation and insufficiency of the (systemic) tricuspid valve (90%), VSD (75%), valvular or subvalvular pulmonary stenosis (75%).

Imaging Signs

▶ **Modality of choice**
Echocardiography • MRI in older patients.

▶ **Chest radiograph findings**
The cardiac silhouette presents a straight upper left border formed by the ascending aorta • Cardiomegaly • Increased pulmonary vascular markings in patients with a large VSD • Enlargement of the LA • AV insufficiency.

▶ **Echocardiographic and MRI findings**
Systemic veins drain into the RA • Pulmonary veins drain into the LA • Echocardiography and MRI can demonstrate atrioventricular and ventriculoarterial discordance • Vertically placed septum • Discontinuity between the aortic and tricuspid valve rings • Evaluation of cardiac function (especially RV function) • Detection of associated anomalies.

▶ **Invasive diagnostic procedures**
Atrioventricular and ventriculoarterial relationships • Invasive tests may be used to define the coronary system • VSD • RVOT obstruction • Determination of hemodynamic functional parameters.

Clinical Aspects

▶ **Typical presentation**
Patients with isolated levo-TGA may remain asymptomatic until adulthood • Complications often do not appear until 30–40 years of age • Progressive tricuspid insufficiency • Right-sided heart failure • Atrial arrhythmias • AV block.

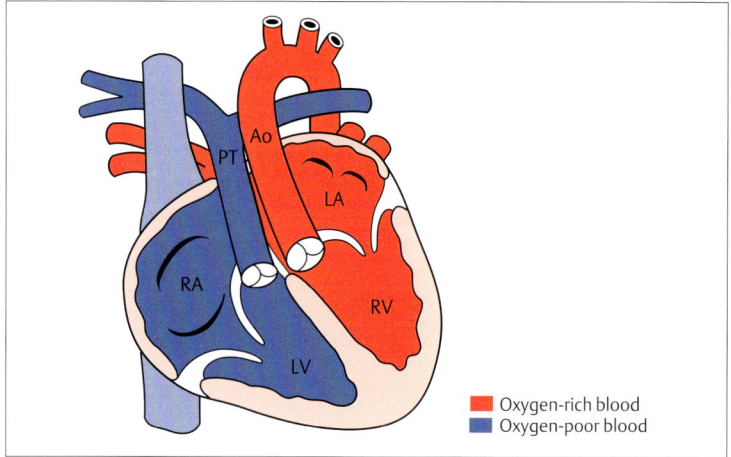

Oxygen-rich blood
Oxygen-poor blood

Fig. 9.38 Diagrammatic illustration of atrioventricular and ventriculoarterial discordance in levo-TGA. The RA drains into the morphologic LV, which is connected to the pulmonary artery. The LA drains into the morphologic RV, from which blood is ejected into the aorta.

▶ **Treatment options**
Medical stabilization of heart failure • Cardiac pacemaker for complete AV block or symptomatic bradycardia.
Surgical options:
– *Double switch:* The morphologic LV becomes the systemic ventricle.
– Combination of atrial switch (Senning or Mustard) and arterial switch.
– Combination of atrial switch (Senning or Mustard) and ventriculoarterial switch (Rastelli; in patients with LVOT obstruction).
Treatment may include the surgical correction of associated anomalies: VSD repair • Pulmonary banding (with a large VSD) • Modified Blalock–Taussig anastomosis (with pulmonary stenosis) • Heart transplantation in rare cases.
Long-term complications: Sinus node dysfunction • Atrial tachyarrhythmias • Baffle stenosis.

▶ **Course and prognosis**
Relative high rate of reoperations • Median life expectancy is 40 years • Life expectancy depends mainly on associated anomalies • Most frequent cause of death—sudden cardiac death, heart failure.

▶ **What does the clinician want to know?**
Signs of heterotaxia • Coexisting anomalies.

Differential Diagnosis

VSD, double-outlet ventricle, tricuspid atresia	– Heart failure – Increased pulmonary blood flow
TOF	– Cyanosis – Decreased pulmonary blood flow

Selected References

Borth-Bruns T, Eichler A (eds.). Pädiatrische Kardiologie. Berlin, Heidelberg: Springer; 2004

Bove EL. Congenitally corrected transposition of the great arteries: ventricle to pulmonary artery connection strategies. Semin Thorac Cardiovasc Surg 1995; 7: 139–144

Gaudio C et al. Therapeutic assessment of adult patients with isolated corrected transposition of the great arteries. G Ital Cardiol 1998; 28: 714–717

Kumpf M, Borth-Bruns T, Nollert G. Angeborene Herzfehler. In: Mewis C, Riessen R, Spyridopoulos I (eds.). Kardiologie compact. Stuttgart: Thieme; 2004

Warnes CA. Transposition of the great arteries. Circulation 2006; 114: 2699–2709

Definition

▶ **Definition, epidemiology**
Ventriculoarterial connection that includes various cardiac anomalies from a clinical and hemodynamic point of view • 0.6–1.5% of all congenital cardiac anomalies.

▶ **Pathoanatomy**
DORV is usually marked by concordant atrioventricular connections (the RA drains into the RV, the LA into the LV) • Both the aorta and pulmonary trunk arise entirely or predominantly from the RV • Variable anatomic relationships • Frequent presence of associated vascular anomalies (coarctation of the aorta, subpulmonary stenosis) • Interventricular connection through a large VSD • Anomalous coronary origins • Positional anomalies of the impulse conduction system.

Imaging Signs

▶ **Modality of choice**
Echocardiography • MRI in older patients.

▶ **Chest radiograph findings**
Cardiomegaly • Increased pulmonary vascular markings in the absence of pulmonary stenosis.

▶ **Echocardiographic and MRI findings**
Precise morphologic analysis • Aorta and pulmonary trunk arise from the RV • Location and size of the VSD • RVOT obstruction • LVOT obstruction • ASD • coarctation of the aorta • Determination of flow volumes in the pulmonary and systemic circulations • Shunt volumes • Ventricular function.

▶ **Invasive diagnostic procedures**
Strict selection criteria should be applied • May be done to measure the pressure gradient across an outflow tract stenosis • Pressure in the pulmonary circulation • Coronary angiography to check for coronary anomalies (other options are MRI and multidetector CT).

Clinical Aspects

▶ **Typical presentation**
Symptoms depend on the anatomic configuration of the anomaly • The dominant feature may be cyanosis or heart failure.

▶ **Treatment options**
Patients with critical pulmonary stenosis can be given prostaglandin E_1 to keep the ductus arteriosus patent until a shunt is implanted • Endocarditis prophylaxis • Rashkind maneuver may be indicated in patients with a restrictive interatrial connection and subpulmonary VSD ($SaO_2 < 70\%$) • Surgical treatment is like that for dextro-TGA or TOF, depending on anatomy.

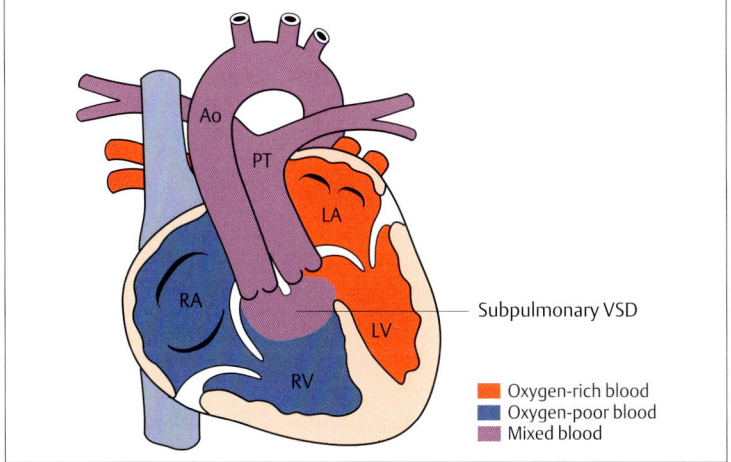

Subpulmonary VSD

■ Oxygen-rich blood
■ Oxygen-poor blood
■ Mixed blood

Fig. 9.39 Diagrammatic illustration of double-outlet right ventricle (DORV). The aorta and pulmonary artery arise from the right ventricle. DORV here is associated with a subpulmonary VSD.

▶ **Course and prognosis**
The mortality rate of corrective operations is approximately 5–15 % ● The 15-year survival rate is 90–95 % ● Supraventricular and ventricular arrhythmias may develop after surgery.

▶ **What does the clinician want to know?**
Location and size of the VSD ● Subpulmonary or subaortic outflow tract obstruction ● ASD ● Coronary anomalies ● Abnormal mitral valve ● Ventricular size and function.

Differential Diagnosis
....

TOF   – Overriding aorta
                           – Similar clinical presentation

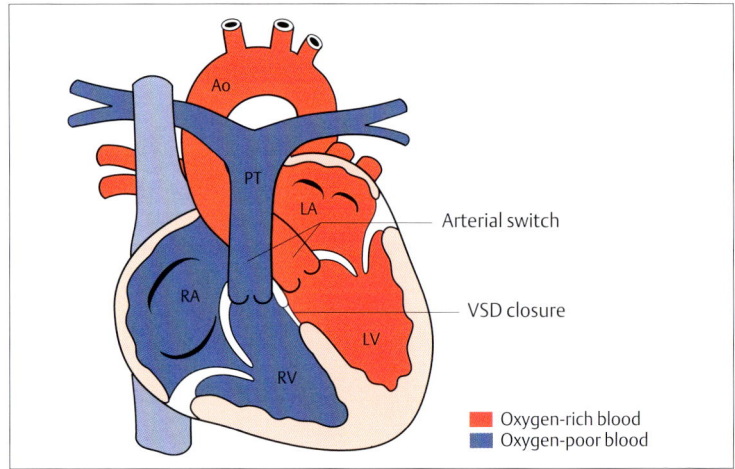

Fig. 9.40 The goal of early surgical treatment in DORV is to achieve a definitive correction. The aorta is connected to the LV, the pulmonary artery to the RV. The VSD is closed.

Tips and Pitfalls

DORV can be difficult to distinguish from TOF in some cases • This differentiation may require further investigation by MRI.

Selected References

Anderson RH et al. Continuing medical education. Double outlet right ventricle. Cardiol Young 2001; 11: 329–344

Borth-Bruns T, Eichler A (eds.). Pädiatrische Kardiologie. Berlin, Heidelberg: Springer; 2004

Lacour-Gayet F. Biventricular repair of double outlet right ventricle with noncommitted ventricular septal defect. Semin Thorac Cardiovasc Surg Pediatr Card Surg Annu 2002; 5: 163–172

Niezen RA et al. Double outlet right ventricle assessed with magnetic resonance imaging. Int J Card Imaging 1999; 15: 323–329

Definition

▶ **Epidemiology**
Rare congenital heart defect (approximately 1%).

▶ **Pathoanatomy, pathophysiology**
All four pulmonary veins drain into systemic veins or into the RA ● Compatible with life only if an intracardiac right-to-left shunt is present (usually a PFO) ● Increased pulmonary blood flow ● 30% of patients have pulmonary venous obstruction with subsequent pulmonary congestion ● This causes a rise in pulmonary arterial pressure ● The retrocardiac collecting vein may have a supra-, intra- or infracardiac termination.

Imaging Signs

▶ **Modality of choice**
Echocardiography for initial evaluation ● MRI or CT for postoperative evaluation.

▶ **Chest radiograph findings**
Findings range from a narrow cardiac silhouette and mediastinum to cardiomegaly, depending on the termination type ● Pulmonary venous obstruction leads to increased pulmonary markings on the chest film ● Edema.

▶ **Echocardiographic findings**
No connection between the pulmonary veins and LA ● Possible RA and RV enlargement ● PFO ● Detection of associated anomalies ● Limited ability to evaluate the proximal pulmonary veins in postoperative patients ● MRI or CT is preferred after surgery.

▶ **CT findings**
Useful before and after surgery ● Can be used to determine pulmonary venous diameters ● Detection of anastomotic stenosis ● Signs of pulmonary congestion (thickened interlobar septa, peribronchial edema, ground-glass opacity).

▶ **MRI findings**
Same as echocardiography and CT findings ● Contrast-enhanced MRA shows no connection between the pulmonary veins and LA ● May show enlargement of the RA and RV ● Visualization of the PFO ● Evaluation of cardiac function ● Valvular insufficiency ● Associated cardiac anomalies.

▶ **Invasive diagnostic procedures**
Rarely necessary in the initial workup ● May be done postoperatively for the detection and interventional treatment of pulmonary venous stenosis.

Clinical Aspects

▶ **Typical presentation**
Depends on the degree of pulmonary venous obstruction and the interatrial connection:
– *No significant obstruction:* Tachypnea ● Heart failure ● Growth retardation.
– *Severe obstruction:* Emergency situation ● Respiratory distress ● Cyanosis.

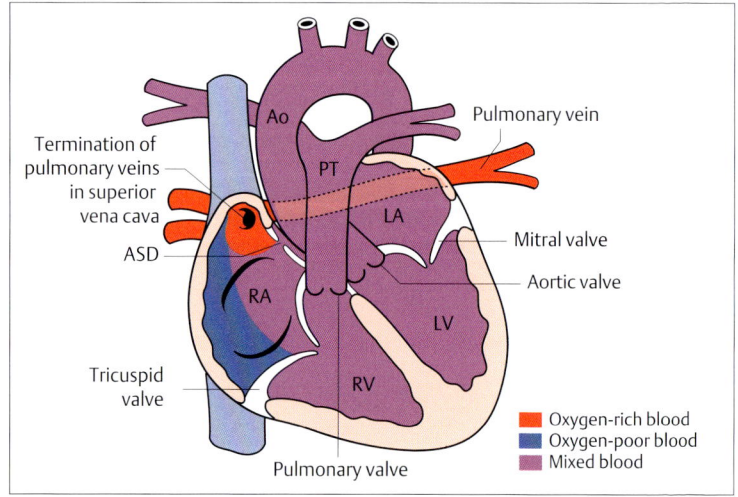

Fig. 9.41 Diagrammatic illustration of TAPVC. All four pulmonary veins drain into the superior vena cava (type I), producing an extracardiac left-to-right shunt. Mixed blood flows into the LA through an ASD.

▶ **Treatment options**

Affected newborns may require immediate corrective surgery under emergency conditions.

Aftercare: Endocarditis prophylaxis • Long-term follow-up for the development of pulmonary vein stenosis (5–10%) and atrial tachycardia following repair of TAPVC.

▶ **Course and prognosis**

Good prognosis after successful surgical repair.

▶ **What does the clinician want to know?**

Type of pulmonary venous termination • Pulmonary vascular status • Signs of congestion • Associated cardiac anomalies • ASD, PFO • Pressure values in the pulmonary circulation.

Differential Diagnosis

Cor triatriatum	– Pulmonary veins drain into the LA
HLHS	– Hypoplasia and obstruction of the LV and LVOT
	– Blood from pulmonary veins enters the RA through the foramen ovale
	– Systemic perfusion through a PDA

Tips and Pitfalls

Occasionally, spin-echo sequences (MRI) are of limited value for delineating the pulmonary venous wall • Contrast-enhanced multidetector CT, SSFP sequences, and contrast-enhanced MRA are better for the detection of anastomotic stenosis.

Selected References

Ashoush R et al. Total anomalous pulmonary venous connection in adults—a surgical review. J Med Liban 1993; 41: 230–235

Kanter KR. Surgical repair of total anomalous pulmonary venous connection. Semin Thorac Cardiovasc Surg Pediatr Card Surg Annu 2006; 40–44

Kumpf M, Borth-Bruns T, Nollert G. Angeborene Herzfehler. In: Mewis C, Riessen R, Spyridopoulos I (eds.). Kardiologie compact. Stuttgart: Thieme; 2004

Lodge AJ et al. Improving outcomes in functional single ventricle and total anomalous pulmonary venous connection. Ann Thorac Surg 2004; 78: 1688–1695

Reddy SC et al. Mixed-type total anomalous pulmonary venous connection: echocardiographic limitations and angiographic advantages. Am Heart J 1995; 129: 1034–1038

Ryerson L, Harder J. Totally anomalous pulmonary venous return. Cardiol Young 2005; 15: 304–305

Definition

▶ **Definition**

Intermediate- or long-term palliative correction of severe congenital heart defects with an anatomic or functional univentricular circulation or of complex anomalies that are not correctible by biventricular surgery • Systemic blood is routed directly to the pulmonary artery, bypassing the subpulmonary ventricle • This procedure separates the circulations and relieves cyanosis.

▶ **Indications**

Heart defects characterized by an anatomic or functional univentricular circulation, i.e., anomalies in which only one ventricle is present or a second ventricle is present but is hypoplastic.
– HLHS.
– Double-outlet left ventricle.
– Aortic or pulmonary atresia without VSD.
– Mitral or tricuspid atresia.
Anomalous termination in one ventricle:
– Double-inlet left ventricle.
– Double-inlet right ventricle.
Uncorrectable malformation of common AV valves:
– AVSD with uncorrectable deformity of the AV valve.

▶ **Principles**

An aortopulmonary shunt is created in the newborn to establish pulmonary perfusion • Not necessary in all forms.
Bidirectional cavopulmonary connection (Glenn operation): This procedure, scheduled at approximately 6 months of age (lower pulmonary resistance), partially separates the circulations • The upper part of the superior vena cava is anastomosed end-to-side to the right pulmonary artery • This reduces the work load on the single ventricle (Q_p:Q_s = 0.6–0.7, PaO_2 = 75–85%).
Fontan procedure after 1–2 years of age: Completely separates the heart into two circulations • The inferior vena cava is connected to the right pulmonary artery, bypassing the RV.
Selection criteria for Fontan palliation: Pulmonary arterial resistance less than twice the upper normal value • Sufficiently large pulmonary arteries without stenosis • Good ventricular function • No severe AV valvular insufficiency • No severe subaortic stenosis.

▶ **Course and prognosis**

Approximately 90% 10-year survival rate in uncomplicated cases • Protein loss and enteropathy are two factors that critically influence postoperative mortality.
– Reoperations are associated with a high mortality (up to 75%).
Late postoperative problems: Atrial flutter or fibrillation • Bradyarrhythmias (sinus node dysfunction, complete AV block) • Thromboembolism • Heart failure due to malformations or stenoses in the Fontan circulation or incompetence of the systemic AV valves • Protein loss or enteropathy (in approximately 10–50% of patients) • Hepatic dysfunction • Cyanosis due to deterioration of ventricular function or right-to-left shunting through the atrial septum.

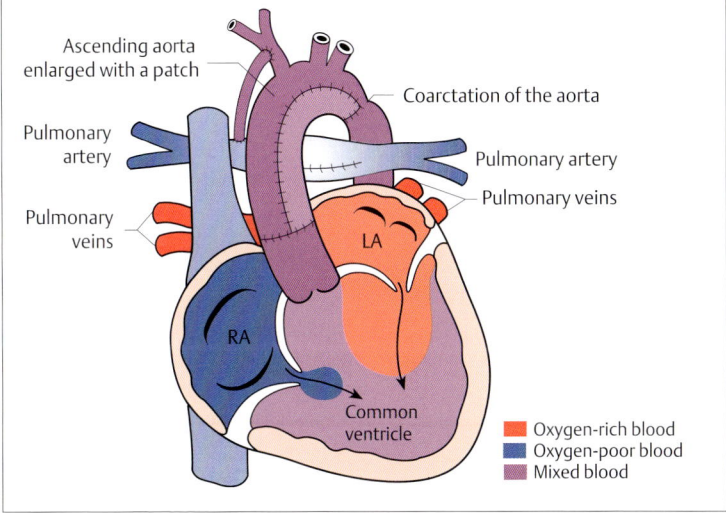

Fig. 9.42 Fontan procedure, Norwood I (illustrated for a univentricular heart). The pulmonary trunk and PDA are divided. The hypoplastic aorta is enlarged with a patch and anastomosed to the pulmonary trunk. A shunt is created between the brachiocephalic trunk and pulmonary artery to direct blood flow to the lung.

▶ **What does the clinician want to know?**
Degree of hypoplasia of the LV and aorta • Size of the PDA and ASD • Ventricular function • Tricuspid insufficiency • Coronary anomalies • Some clinicians may request quantitative evaluation of the pulmonary vascular bed (Nakata index, McGoon ratio), ventricular function, and AV valvular function.

Selected References

Borth Bruns T, Eichler A (eds.). Pädiatrische Kardiologie. Berlin, Heidelberg: Springer; 2004

Freedom RM et al. The Fontan procedure: analysis of cohorts and late complications. Cardiol Young 2000; 10: 307–331

Giroud JM, Jacobs JP. Fontan's operation: evolution from a procedure to a process. Cardiol Young 2006; 16 Suppl 1: 67–71

Jacobs ML, Pelletier G. Late complications associated with the Fontan circulation. Cardiol Young 2006; 16 Suppl 1: 80–84

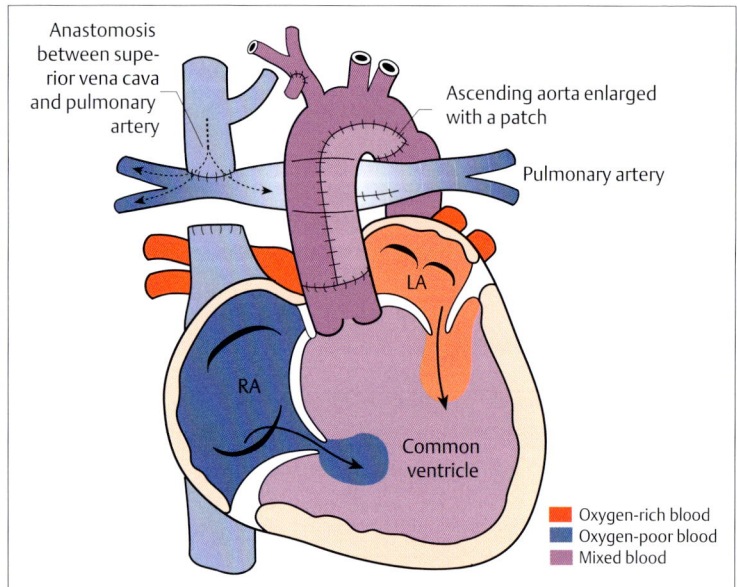

Fig. 9.43 Fontan procedure, Norwood II. The superior vena cava is connected to the right pulmonary artery (Glenn shunt). The shunt between the brachiocephalic trunk and pulmonary artery is divided. This allows pure venous blood to enter the lung, while mixed blood is still present in the systemic circulation.

Jacobs ML, Pourmoghadam KK. The hemi-Fontan operation. Semin Thorac Cardiovasc Surg Pediatr Card Surg Annu 2003; 6: 90–97

Kurosawa H. Current strategies of the Fontan operation. Ann Thorac Cardiovasc Surg 1998; 4: 171–177

Setty SP, Herrington CS. Fontan procedure: old lessons and new frontiers. Expert Rev Cardiovasc Ther 2006; 4: 515–521

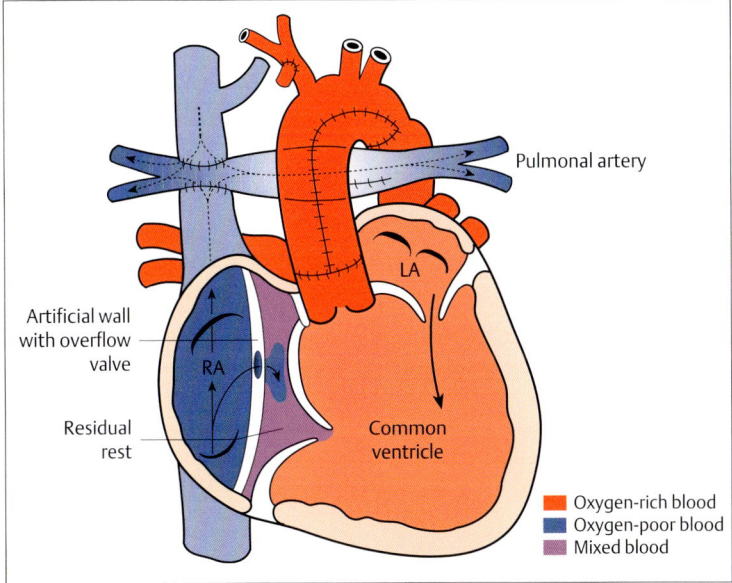

Fig. 9.44 Fontan procedure, Norwood III. The inferior vena cava is connected to the right or left pulmonary artery (Fontan shunt), here by way of an intracardiac tunnel. The tunnel passes through the RA, which is partitioned by a surgically constructed wall. An opening in the patch functions as an "overflow valve" that empties into the residual RA

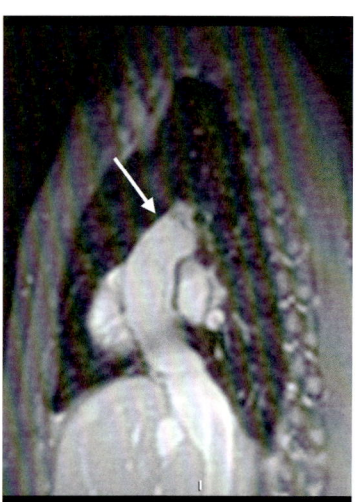

Fig. 9.45 Sagittal MPR of a 3D data set after a Fontan procedure. The image shows the Fontan shunt (inferior vena cava, arrow) connected to the right pulmonary artery.

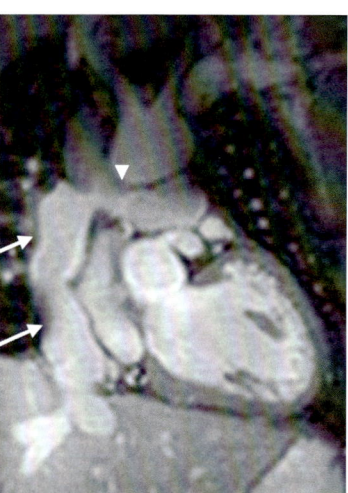

Fig. 9.46 Coronal MPR of a 3D data set after a Fontan procedure. The Fontan shunt (inferior vena cava, arrows) is connected to the right pulmonary artery (arrowhead).

Definition

▶ **Epidemiology**
A palliative procedure • Improves blood flow to the lungs • Reduces cyanosis • *Indications:* TOF, hypoplastic pulmonary arteries, hypoplastic valve ring • Today, few adults are selected for a palliative operation.

▶ **Anatomy**
Two variants of the operation are distinguished:
– *Original Blalock–Taussig shunt:* end-to-side anastomosis between the subclavian artery and pulmonary artery.
– *Modified Blalock–Taussig shunt:* side-to-side anastomosis interposing a PTFE prosthesis between the subclavian artery and pulmonary artery.

Imaging Signs

▶ **Modality of choice**
Echocardiography in small children • MRI in adolescents and adults.

▶ **Echocardiographic findings**
Position and patency of the shunt • If necessary, continuous-wave or color Doppler can be used to determine the flow volume • Visualization of the underlying defect.

▶ **MRI findings**
Same as echocardiographic findings • Image quality improves with age • Morphologic visualization with T1-weighted TSE or SSFP sequence • Contrast-enhanced MRA if required • Flowmetry (phase-contrast imaging) for quantification of the shunt volume.

▶ **Invasive diagnostic procedures**
Rarely indicated • Invasive tests may be done before reoperation for pressure measurements and shunt evaluation.

Clinical Aspects

▶ **Treatment options**
The Blalock–Taussig shunt is designed to improve lung perfusion and oxygenation in patients with cyanotic heart defects.

▶ **Course and prognosis**
Problems after the Blalock–Taussig shunt: shunt occlusion, subclavian steal (original Blalock–Taussig shunt) • Patient may "outgrow" the shunt • Risk of endocarditis • Rare reports of heart failure.

▶ **What does the clinician want to know?**
Original or modified Blalock–Taussig shunt • Shunt patency • Shunt volume • Stenosis • Features of underlying congenital heart defect.

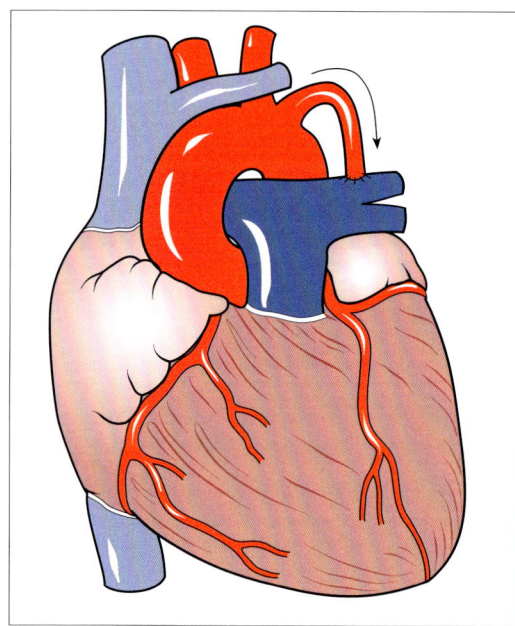

Fig. 9.47 Diagrammatic illustration of a Blalock–Taussig shunt with an end-to-side anastomosis of the left subclavian artery to the left pulmonary artery.

Selected References

Borth-Bruns T, Eichler A (eds.). Pädiatrische Kardiologie. Berlin, Heidelberg: Springer; 2004

Ghanayem NS et al. Right ventricle-to-pulmonary artery conduit versus Blalock-Taussig shunt: a hemodynamic comparison. Ann Thorac Surg 2006; 82: 1603–1609; discussion 1609–1610

Taussig HB et al. Long-time observations of the Blalock-Taussig operation. IV. Tricuspid atresia Johns Hopkins Med J 1973; 132: 135–145

Williams WG et al. Palliation of tricuspid atresia. Potts-Smith, Glenn, and Blalock-Taussig shunts. Arch Surg 1975; 110: 1383–1386

Definition

▶ **Epidemiology**
Thoracic involvement less common than abdominal aortic aneurysm (1:10).

▶ **Definition, pathoanatomy, classification**
Dilatation of an arterial segment to more than 50% its normal diameter (usually 4 cm or more) • Five types are identified in the Crawford classification (see Chapter 12, Appendix).

▶ **Etiology, pathophysiology, pathogenesis**
Aortic aneurysms are usually secondary to atherosclerosis, aortic valve disease, or arterial hypertension • Less common causes are cystic medial necrosis, syphilis, Takayasu arteritis, aortitis, and trauma.

Imaging Signs

▶ **Modality of choice**
CT.

▶ **Chest radiograph findings**
Mediastinal widening • Dilated aortic arch • Aortic configuration of the cardiac silhouette • Aortic sclerosis • Tracheal displacement.

▶ **Echocardiographic findings**
TEE demonstrates the aorta better than TTE • Dilatation of the aorta • Possible aortic valve disease • LV dilatation secondary to aortic insufficiency • Hypertrophy due to aortic stenosis or arterial hypertension.

▶ **CT findings**
Detailed visualization of the aneurysm • Relationship of the aneurysm to the supraaortic vessels • Involvement of the aortic arch (treatment implications) • Plaque formation, ulcerated plaques • Pseudoaneurysms • LV dilatation or hypertrophy.

▶ **MRI findings**
Same as echocardiographic and CT findings • Accurate assessment of ventricular and valvular function • With aortitis, inflammatory changes may be seen on contrast-enhanced MRI.

Clinical Aspects

▶ **Typical presentation**
Asymptomatic for years • Possible swallowing difficulties • Hoarseness • Dyspnea • Back pain • Acute chest pain before or during perforation • Shock due to massive bleeding • Often there is long prior history of arterial hypertension.

▶ **Treatment options**
Antihypertensive therapy • Reconstructive repair (ascending aorta) or prosthetic replacement (descending aorta) • Surgical treatment is indicated for aneurysms larger than 5 cm (ascending aorta) or 6 cm (descending aorta) and for aneurysms growing at a rate of more than 1 cm/year (increasing risk of perforation).

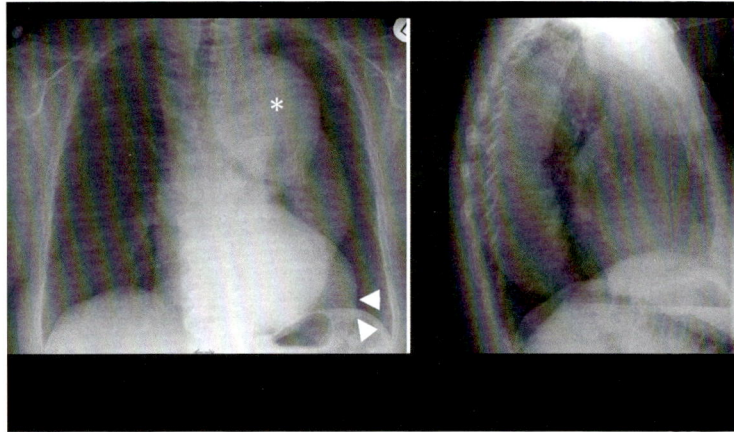

Fig. 10.1   Aortic aneurysm. P-A chest radiograph shows aneurysmal dilatation of the aortic arch to more than 6 cm (*) and marked elongation of the entire thoracic aorta. The cardiac silhouette presents an aortic configuration with a raised apex (arrowheads).

▶ **Course and prognosis**
Frank aneurysms have a 76% spontaneous mortality over a 2-year period • The cause of death in 50% is rupture with acute bleeding • Operated cases have a good prognosis.

▶ **What does the clinician want to know?**
Aortic diameter • Location of the aneurysm • Its relationship to other vessels • Signs of complications (ulcerated plaques and a hyperdense aortic wall are signs of intramural bleeding and impending rupture, pseudoaneurysm, contrast extravasation = bleeding).

Differential Diagnosis

Complications of aneurysms and atherosclerosis: Pseudoaneurysm, aortic dissection or intramural hemorrhage, plaque ulceration.

Tips and Pitfalls

In the age of multidetector CT, MPRs should be obtained and closely scrutinized for the confident detection of complications and early signs of rupture. Unenhanced spiral CT scans should also be obtained in acutely symptomatic patients to detect acute hemorrhage.

Selected References

Yanqing S. Thoracic aortic aneurysm and dissection: surgical results and experience of 428 cases. Heart Lung Circ 2001; 10: A32–33

Definition

▶ **Epidemiology**
Incidence increases with age.

▶ **Etiology, pathophysiology, pathogenesis**
Atherosclerosis • Aortic valve disease • Arterial hypertension • Less common causes are cystic medial necrosis, Marfan and Ehlers–Danlos syndromes, and inflammatory diseases (e.g., syphilis, Takayasu arteritis).

▶ **Pathoanatomy**
The vessel caliber is increased, but by less than 50% of the normal diameter of that aortic segment (e.g., ascending aorta is usually in the range of 3–4 cm).

Imaging Signs

▶ **Modality of choice**
CT.

▶ **Chest radiograph findings**
Often there is nonspecific mediastinal widening • Cardiac contour may be normal • LV enlargement due to aortic insufficiency • Aortic configuration due to aortic stenosis.

▶ **Echocardiographic findings**
Increased diameter of the ascending aorta • Possible aortic insufficiency or stenosis, which determine the degree of severity • Evaluation of LV function.

▶ **CT findings**
CT gives clearest delineation of the thoracic aorta • *Comparison with reference vessels:* The diameter of the ascending aorta in patients with normal pulmonary status should be equal to the diameter of the pulmonary trunk.

▶ **MRI findings**
Same as CT findings • MRI can also evaluate the aortic valve and cardiac function • Aortic valve disease can be quantified if necessary by flowmetry.

Clinical Aspects

▶ **Typical presentation**
Generally asymptomatic • Often detected incidentally.

▶ **Treatment options**
Antihypertensive therapy • Aortic valve replacement may be indicated in patients with aortic stenosis • Regular follow-ups should be scheduled to check for enlargement and development of aneurysms that would necessitate surgery.

▶ **Course and prognosis**
Good prognosis with appropriate therapy and prompt surgical intervention.

▶ **What does the clinician want to know?**
Location and diameter • Progression over time • Changes in the aortic valve.

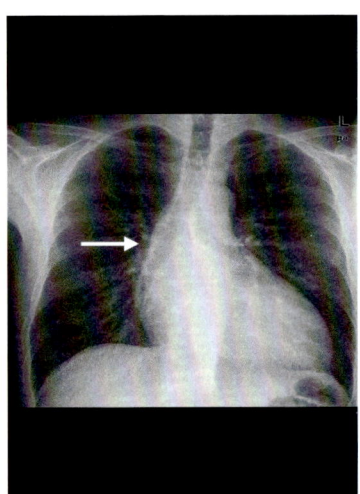

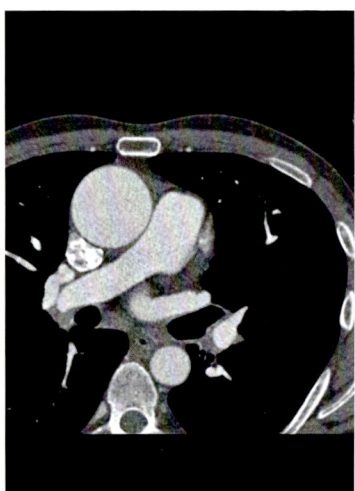

Fig. 10.2 Aortic ectasia in a patient with grade II aortic insufficiency. P-A chest radiograph shows widening of the left cardiac silhouette due to LV dilatation. The ascending aorta forms the right border of the cardiac silhouette.

Fig. 10.3 Same patient as in Fig. 10.**2**. Axial contrast-enhanced thoracic multidetector CT shows dilatation of the ascending aorta to 4 cm. Its diameter is considerably greater than that of the pulmonary trunk. (Normally the diameters of the two vessels should be approximately equal.)

Differential Diagnosis

Aortic aneurysm, other mediastinal masses.

Tips and Pitfalls

If any aortic abnormalities are noted on the chest radiograph, especially in patients with arterial hypertension, echocardiography or CT should be done.

Selected References

Givehchian M et al. Aortic root remodeling: functional MRI as an accurate tool for complete follow-up. Thorac Cardiovasc Surg 2005; 53: 267–273

Kvitting JP et al. Flow patterns in the aortic root and the aorta studied with time-resolved, 3-dimensional, phase-contrast magnetic resonance imaging: implications for aortic valve-sparing surgery. J Thorac Cardiovasc Surg 2004; 127: 1602–1607

Definition

▶ **Epidemiology**
Prevalence of approximately 5200/100 000 in Western countries ● Involves the ascending aorta in approximately two-thirds of cases ● More common in males than in females (3:1).

▶ **Pathoanatomy, classification**
An aortic dissection has a true and a false lumen, the false lumen usually being larger ● The false lumen may completely compress the true lumen, leading to acute ischemia of dependent vascular regions ● Stanford classification (better established clinically) or DeBakey classification.

▶ **Etiology, pathophysiology, pathogenesis**
A tear in the intima leads to progressive subintimal bleeding ("entry") and dissection ● Initial tear results from atheromatous changes in the aortic wall ● Arterial hypertension ● Connective-tissue diseases (Marfan syndrome, Ehlers–Danlos syndrome) ● Inflammatory diseases (giant cell arteritis, Takayasu arteritis, Behçet disease) ● Trauma (thoracic trauma, catheterization) ● Often precipitated by a hypertensive event.

Imaging Signs

▶ **Modality of choice**
TEE, CT if TEE is unavailable.

▶ **Chest radiograph findings**
Mediastinal widening ● Enlarged cardiac silhouette (hemopericardium) ● Pleural effusion due to perforation and hemothorax ● *Caution:* Up to 25% of cases do not have abnormal findings in the chest radiograph.

▶ **Echocardiographic findings**
TEE can demonstrate all relevant findings—intimal flap, aneurysm, aortic valve involvement, acute aortic insufficiency, LV dilatation, coronary dissection, and pericardial effusion.

▶ **CT findings**
Same as echocardiographic findings, but aortic valve function cannot be assessed ● CT can disclose additional sites of vascular involvement (supraaortic, upper abdominal vessels) ● Associated complications (renal and gastrointestinal ischemia) ● May yield better information for planning treatment.

▶ **MRI findings**
Indicated only in patients with chronic dissection ● Same as Echocardiographic and CT findings ● More precise delineation of morphology and functional indicators (aortic valve, ventricular function) ● Particularly useful for follow-up.

Fig. 10.4 Contrast-enhanced thoracic multidetector CT in a 55-year-old man with acute chest pain. Sagittal reconstruction shows an acute type A dissection of the entire thoracic aorta with an intramural hematoma involving part of the ascending aorta. The dissection extends into the abdominal aorta. Opacification of the false lumen (arrows) is delayed relative to the true lumen.

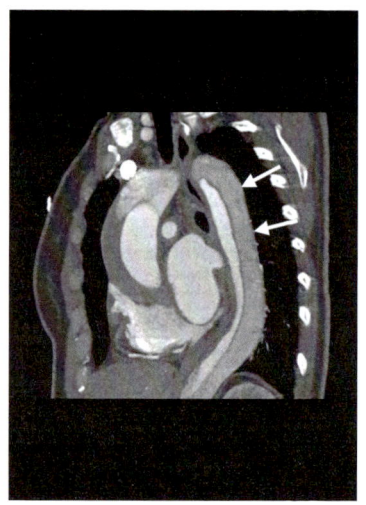

Fig. 10.5 Same patient as in Fig. 10.4. Axial CT scan at the level of the aortic arch shows different contrast characteristics of the true lumen (small arrow) and false lumen (large arrow).

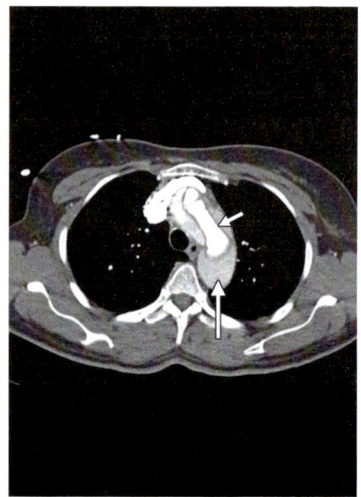

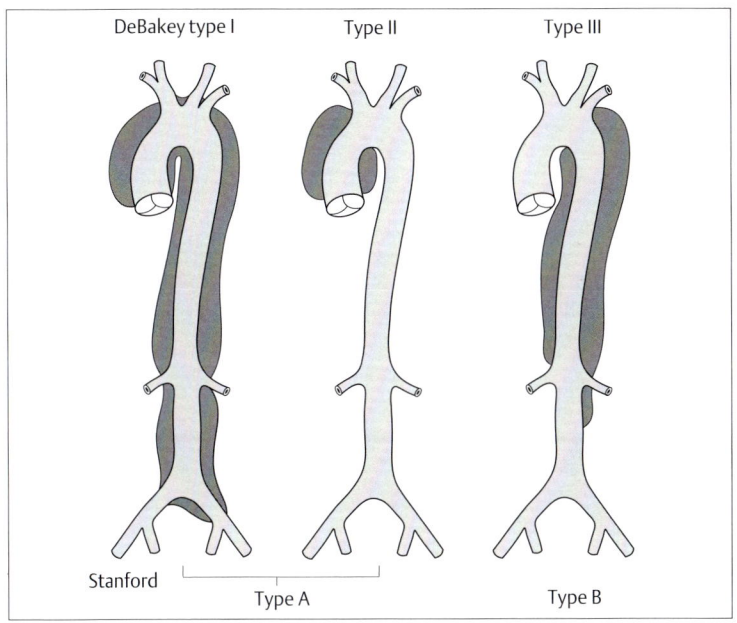

Fig. 10.6 Stanford and DeBakey classifications of aortic dissection.

Stanford type A: Dissection involving the ascending aorta.

Stanford type B: Dissection not involving the ascending aorta.

DeBakey type I: Dissection starts at the ascending aorta and continues into the aortic arch and descending aorta.

DeBakey type II: Involves only the ascending aorta.

DeBakey type III: Starts at the descending aorta and continues distally; very rarely shows retrograde extension into the aortic arch.

Clinical Aspects

▶ **Typical presentation**

Acute: Chest pain of acute onset that radiates to the back • Acute heart failure • Cardiogenic shock in 20% of cases • Spinal cord paralysis.

Chronic: Pulse deficit • Neurologic deficit (progressive paraplegia) • Rarely asymptomatic.

▶ **Treatment options**

Type A: Always a life-threatening emergency • Requires surgicalreplacement of the ascending aorta • May necessitate valve repair or replacement • Reimplantation of the coronary arteries.

Type B: Antihypertensive therapy • Operative treatment after the patient is stabilized • Endovascular stent grafts are implanted in patients with acute bleeding • Percutaneous fenestration of the intimal flap is recommended in patients with peripheral ischemia.

▶ **Course and prognosis**
Type A: Always life-threatening • Up to a 30% 24-hour mortality.
Type B: Conservative therapy has a better prognosis than immediate surgery (3-year survival rate of 95%).

▶ **What does the clinician want to know?**
Location and extent of the dissection • Involvement of supraaortic vessels • Location of the entry and reentry points • Perfusion of the true and false lumina • Secondary complications (pleural effusion, mediastinal hematoma, pericardial tamponade, renal or visceral ischemia).

Differential Diagnosis
....

Acute myocardial infarction • Pulmonary embolism • Aortic rupture • Mesenteric infarction • Perforated ulcer.

Selected References

Hsu RB et al. Outcome of medical and surgical treatment in patients with acute type B aortic dissection. Ann Thorac Surg 2005; 79: 790–794

Nienaber CA et al. The diagnosis of thoracic aortic dissection by noninvasive imaging procedures. N Engl J Med 1993; 328: 1–9

Sullivan PR et al. Diagnosis of acute thoracic aortic dissection in the emergency department. Am J Emerg Med 2000; 18: 46–50

Definition

▶ **Epidemiology**
Prevalence of approximately 3% in the elderly population • Stenosis of the internal carotid artery is responsible for cerebral ischemic attacks in approximately 20% of cases.

▶ **Etiology, pathophysiology, pathogenesis**
Soft or calcified atherosclerotic plaques of the vessel wall lead to a functionally significant stenosis • Risk factors include hypertension, diabetes mellitus, smoking, hypercholesterolemia, genetic predisposition • Typical sites of occurrence are the bulb of the common carotid artery and the proximal third of the internal carotid artery.

Imaging Signs

▶ **Modality of choice**
Color Doppler ultrasound.

▶ **Color Doppler ultrasound findings**
Intimal thickening • Narrowing of the vessel lumen at the stenosis • Systolic flow acceleration • Soft or calcified plaques.

▶ **CT and MRI findings**
Multidetector CT or MR angiography can accurately define the stenosis • Flow acceleration on phase-contrast angiography (MRI) • Along with the history, cerebral MRI can supply information on prior ischemic events (FLAIR sequence may show signs of very small cerebral infarctions).

▶ **Invasive diagnostic procedures**
DSA is generally used when planning interventional stent insertions.

Clinical Aspects

▶ **Typical presentation**
Asymptomatic in 5% of patients • TIAs or stroke (headache, impaired consciousness, neurologic deficits, sensorimotor hemiparesis).

▶ **Treatment options**
Patients with clinical symptoms or greater than 60% stenosis can be treated by thromboendarterectomy • Another option is stent implantation • Regular follow ups are indicated for lesions with less than 60% luminal narrowing • Long-term aspirin treatment is recommended.

▶ **Course and prognosis**
Prognosis is related to the progression of systemic atherosclerosis • Rate of cerebral ischemic attacks is markedly reduced after therapy.

▶ **What does the clinician want to know?**
Location and degree of the stenosis • Plaque morphology • Other lesions of the supraaortic vessels.

Fig. 10.7 Carotid stenosis. B-mode ultrasound demonstrates a localized, eccentric, calcified plaque at the carotid bifurcation. The plaque casts an acoustic shadow (arrow) (from Kubale R, Stiegler H. *Farbkodierte Duplexsonographie*. Stuttgart: Thieme, 2002). ACC, common carotid artery; ACE, external carotid artery; ACI, internal carotid artery.

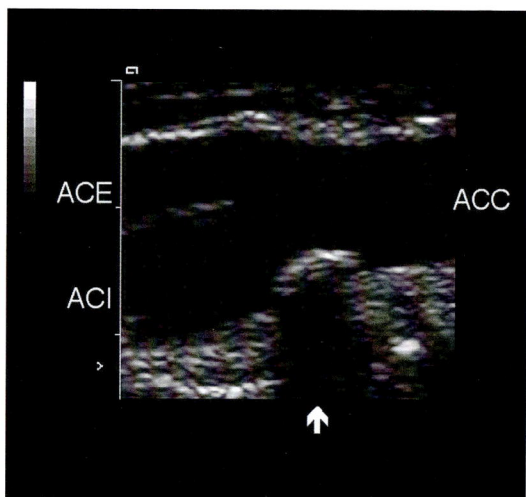

Fig. 10.8 Contrast-enhanced MRA. MIP reveals high-grade proximal stenosis of both internal carotid arteries, moderate stenosis of the left subclavian artery, and plaque stenosis of the brachiocephalic trunk (arrows).

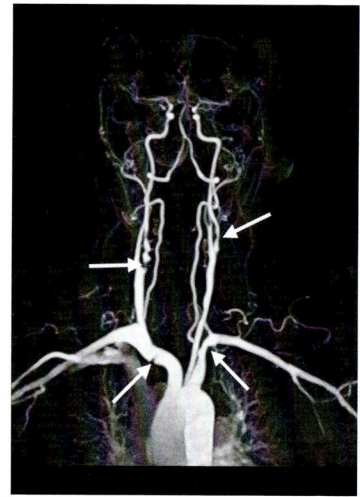

Differential Diagnosis

Carotid dissection • Vascular compression by a glomus tumor • Branchial cleft cyst • Lymphoma • Goiter • Other masses.

Tips and Pitfalls

The degree of stenosis is often overestimated by MRA (e.g., a subtotal stenosis interpreted as a pseudo-occlusion) • Thus, the preoperative MRA diagnosis of an occlusion should always be checked with another modality (color Doppler ultrasound, DSA) • Always examine both sides, as occasionally there is bilateral stenosis.

Selected References

Chaturvedi S et al. Therapeutics and Technology Assessment Subcommittee of the American Academy of Neurology. Carotid endarterectomy – an evidence-based review: report of the Therapeutics and Technology Assessment Subcommittee of the American Academy of Neurology. Neurology 2005; 65: 794–801

Edward G et al. Carotid Artery Stenosis: Gray-Scale and Doppler US Diagnosis Society of Radiologists in Ultrasound Consensus Conference. Radiology 2003; 229: 340–346

Definition

▶ **Epidemiology**

A rare, generally acquired cause of TIA • More common in males that in females (3:1) • Predisposition for left subclavian artery (four times more common than the right) • 80% of patients have concomitant atherosclerotic changes in the cervical vessels.

▶ **Etiology, pathophysiology, pathogenesis**

Atherosclerotic, congenital, or secondary to vasculitis • High-grade stenosis or occlusion of the proximal subclavian artery proximal to the origin of the vertebral artery • With strenuous arm exercise, collateral blood flow reverses the direction of flow in the vertebral artery, which steals blood from the circle of Willis, causing cerebral ischemia.

Imaging Signs

▶ **Modality of choice**

Continuous-wave Doppler • Color Doppler ultrasound.

▶ **Color Doppler ultrasound findings**

Flow reversal in the vertebral artery on the affected side • This phenomenon is increased by arm exercise • May demonstrate the subclavian stenosis in some cases.

▶ **CT and MRI findings**

Precise angiographic visualization of the stenosis or occlusion on postcontrast images (CTA, MRA) • May disclose additional vascular lesions (carotid artery, brachiocephalic trunk) • Phase-contrast angiography (MRI) can demonstrate reversal of flow in the vertebral artery.

▶ **Invasive diagnostic procedures**

DSA is obsolete as a diagnostic tool • Angiography is still used in planning interventional therapy and at times for determining pre- and postinterventional pressure gradients.

Clinical Aspects

▶ **Typical presentation**

Often asymptomatic • Syncopal attacks • Nausea • Vertigo • TIA or PRIND • Pulse deficit, weakness and sensory disturbances in the affected limb • Symptoms are exacerbated by arm exercise.

▶ **Treatment options**

The primary options are interventional balloon angioplasty and stent implantation • Another option is bypass surgery.

▶ **Course and prognosis**

Good prognosis after successful treatment • Rate of 5-year patency after stent implantation is higher than 85%.

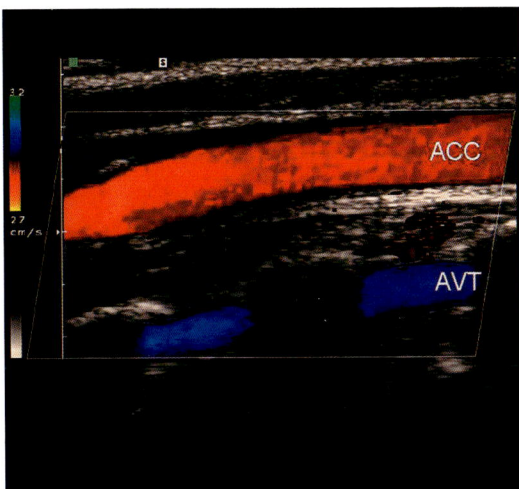

Fig. 10.9 Permanent subclavian steal effect. Color Doppler demonstrates retrograde flow in the vertebral artery (AVT), opposite to the direction of flow in the common carotid artery (ACC) (from Kubale R, Stiegler H. *Farbkodierte Duplexsonographie*. Stuttgart: Thieme, 2002).

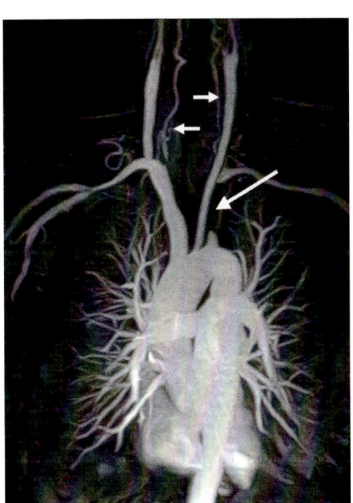

Fig. 10.10 Subclavian artery. MIP from a contrast-enhanced MR angiographic study shows an occlusion of the left subclavian artery proximal to the origin of the vertebral artery (large arrow). The patent vertebral artery is clearly visualized on both sides (small arrows).

▶ **What does the clinician want to know?**
Location and length of the stenosis or occlusion of the subclavian artery • Collateralization • Flow reversal in the vertebral artery • Additional stenoses of the supraaortic vessels (especially the carotid artery).

Differential Diagnosis

Occlusion or stenosis of the brachiocephalic trunk	– Steal syndrome involving the right carotid artery
Carotid dissection, vascular compression	– Tumor – Trauma
Vertebrobasilar insufficiency	– Cerebrovascular disease or organic brain disease

Tips and Pitfalls

Occlusion of the superior vena cava is occasionally detected incidentally (in up to 3% of older patients with symptomatic atherosclerosis) • The finding should be noted and the patient referred for further testing.

Selected References

Bitar R et al. MR angiography of subclavian steal syndrome: pitfalls and solutions. AJR Am J Roentgenol 2004; 183: 1840–1841

De Vries JP et al. Durability of percutaneous transluminal angioplasty for obstructive lesions of proximal subclavian artery: long-term results. J Vasc Surg 2005; 41: 19–23

Definition

▶ **Epidemiology**
   Peak incidence at 20–50 years of age • More common in females than in males (3:1).

▶ **Etiology, pathophysiology, pathogenesis**
   Syndrome caused by compression of the neurovascular bundle in the thoracic outlet • The brachial plexus and the subclavian artery and vein may be compressed by a cervical rib or atypical first rib (congenital), by excessive fracture callus formation or exostosis of the first rib (acquired), and in rare cases by muscular hypertrophy or fibrosis (scalene muscles) or a tumor • Compression of the brachial plexus is much more common than entrapment of the subclavian artery (TOS) or the subclavian vein (thoracic inlet syndrome).

Imaging Signs

▶ **Modality of choice**
   MRA.

▶ **Chest radiograph findings**
   Normal cardiopulmonary findings • May demonstrate a cervical rib • May show callus formation after a clavicular fracture • May demonstrate fracture or exostosis of the first rib.

▶ **CT findings**
   Not indicated because the patient must be examined at rest and during a provocative maneuver.

▶ **MRI findings**
   MRA shows focal occlusion of the subclavian artery during hyperabduction of the arms • The venous system is examined in the same way during the venous phase.

▶ **Invasive diagnostic procedures**
   Intraarterial DSA is no longer indicated • Although outdated, intravenous DSA can be done through a central venous line for examining the patient at rest and during a provocative maneuver • If stenosis or thrombosis of the subclavian vein is suspected, venography is carried out through the ipsilateral venous system.

Clinical Aspects

▶ **Typical presentation**
   Symptoms typically appear during overhead work—pain • Paresthesias • Muscular atrophy • Raynaud syndrome • Claudication • Pulse deficit • Thrombosis (usually venous).

▶ **Treatment options**
   Physical therapy • Some cases may require surgical decompression by resection of the cervical rib or first rib or by a scalene plasty.

▶ **Course and prognosis**
   Very good • Patients remain asymptomatic in 80–100% of cases.

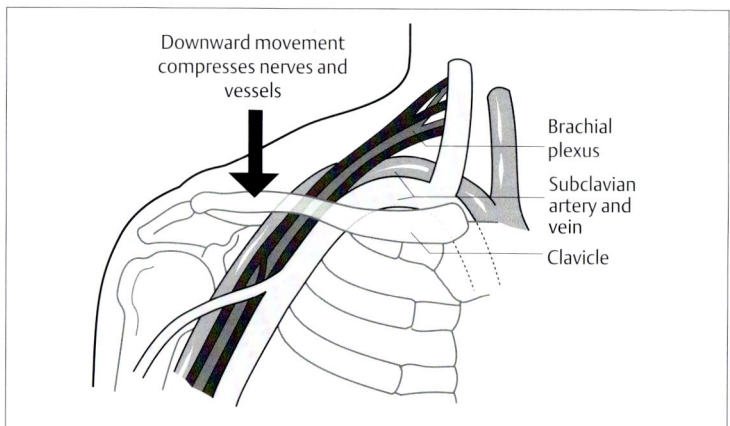

Fig. 10.11 Anatomy of thoracic outlet syndrome. Besides compression by a cervical rib, the subclavian artery may become entrapped beneath the clavicle or in the interscalene triangle. Compression of the brachial plexus is much more common than entrapment of the subclavian artery (TOS) or the subclavian vein (thoracic inlet syndrome).

Fig. 10.12 a, b
Intravenous DSA at rest and during a provocative maneuver (raising the right arm and turning the head to the left). Film at rest (**a**) demonstrates a normal caliber of the right subclavian artery. Film during the provocative maneuver (**b**) shows an abrupt cutoff of the contrast column (arrow) due to vascular compression, caused in this case by a cervical rib.

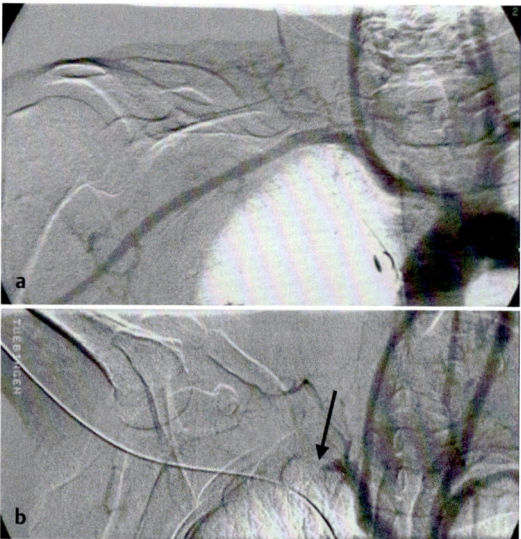

▶ **What does the clinician want to know?**
Site of the vascular compression • Complete occlusion • Anatomic variant (cervical rib, old fracture) • Thrombosis • Contralateral findings.

Differential Diagnosis

Neurologic diseases	– Cervical radiculopathy
	– Reflex sympathetic dystrophy
	– Plexus injuries
Vascular diseases	– Aneurysm
	– Thromboembolism
	– Vasculitis (Raynaud disease)
Masses	– Pancoast tumor
	– Compression by hematoma

Tips and Pitfalls

MRA with i.v. contrast administration at the ipsilateral elbow may yield poor imaging results due to venous stasis.

Selected References

Charon JP et al. Evaluation of MR angiographic technique in the assessment of thoracic outlet syndrome. Clin Radiol 2004; 59: 588–595

McSweeney SE et al. Thoracic outlet syndrome secondary to first rib anomaly: the value of multi-slice CT in diagnosis and surgical planning. Ir Med J 2005; 98: 246–247

Definition

▶ **Epidemiology**
Rare disease (prevalence of 1–3 per million) • Most common in Asians, with an 8:1 female preponderance • Initial symptoms appear before age 30 in 80% of cases.

▶ **Etiology, pathophysiology, pathogenesis**
Granulomatous vasculitis, probably autoimmune mediated • Predominantly affects the major arteries, especially the aorta and its branches, as well as pulmonary and coronary arteries • Proliferative fibrotic changes in the tunica media lead to segmental stenoses, occlusions, or aneurysms.

Imaging Signs

▶ **Modality of choice**
MRI.

▶ **Chest radiograph findings**
Normal cardiopulmonary findings.

▶ **Color Doppler ultrasound**
Wall thickening • Vascular stenosis • Increased systolic flow velocity in accessible vascular regions (supraaortic, cervical, temporal and mesenteric arteries).

▶ **PET, PET, and CT findings**
Increased FDG uptake in the inflamed vascular segment • FDG uptake can be evaluated to assess therapeutic response.

▶ **MRI findings**
Contrast enhancement • Increased T2-weighted signal intensity • Circumscribed wall thickening (> 3 mm) of the aorta and its branches • MRI often shows smooth, long-segment stenoses or occlusions • Aneurysms and thrombi • Collateral vessels.

▶ **CT findings**
Findings same as MRI • Less sensitive.

▶ **Invasive diagnostic procedures**
Conventional angiography is used mainly for planning interventional procedures and examining small vessels (e.g., coronary angiography).

Clinical Aspects

▶ **Typical presentation**
Acute inflammation • Fever • Pain in affected arteries • Subsequent vascular occlusions • Aneurysms • Aortic dissection • Hypertension • Neurologic deficit • Intestinal ischemia.

▶ **Treatment options**
High-dose steroid therapy (necessary in up to 60% of cases) • Immunosuppressants (methotrexate and cyclophosphamide) may also be beneficial • Vascular stenoses are treated by interventional or surgical therapy.

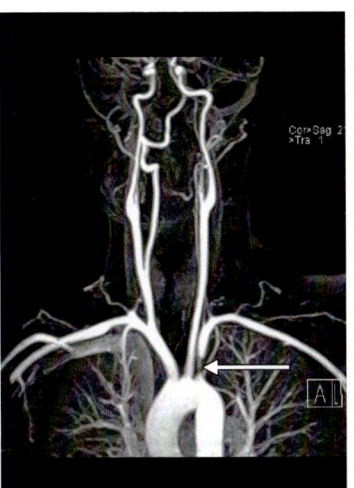

Fig. 10.13 Contrast-enhanced MRA of Takayasu arteritis in a 42-year-old woman. MIP shows proximal stenosis of the subclavian artery (arrow) caused by inflammatory wall changes.

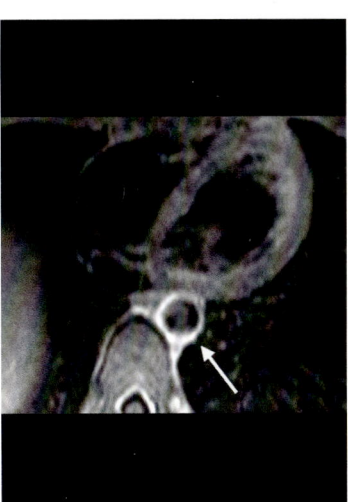

Fig. 10.14 Same patient as in Fig. 10.**13**. Axial T1-weighted TSE sequence after gadolinium-DTPA administration demonstrates wall thickening and marked enhancement of the descending aorta (arrow).

▶ **Course and prognosis**

Most untreated cases have a fatal outcome (death due to myocardial infarction and stroke) • Involvement of the carotid artery causes neurologic symptoms in 80% of patients (TIAs, stroke) • Patients are often free of complaints with appropriate therapy • 10-year survival rate is approximately 90%.

▶ **What does the clinician want to know?**

Location of stenoses and inflamed wall segments.

Differential Diagnosis

Giant-cell arteritis (predominantly affects medium-sized vessels such as the temporal artery), other forms of vasculitis (panarteritis nodosa, Winiwarter–Buerger disease), and collagen diseases.

Tips and Pitfalls

Do not overlook a systemic component with an acute inflammatory reaction in the vessel wall or additional, previously asymptomatic, manifestations.

Selected References

Fritz J et al. Current imaging in Takayasu arteritis. Fortschr Röntgenstr 2005; 177: 1467–1472

Kerr GS et al. Takayasu arteritis. Ann Intern Med 1994; 120: 919–929

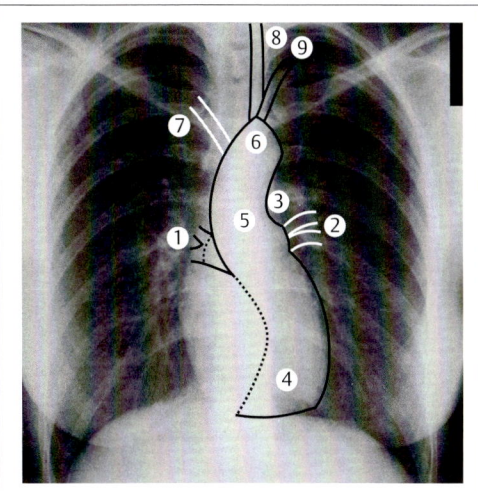

Fig. 11.1 Left cardiac structures and major vessels:
1 Right upper lobe vein
2 Left upper lobe vein
3 Left atrial appendage
4 Left ventricle
5 Ascending aorta
6 Aortic arch
7 Brachiocephalic trunk
8 Left common carotid artery
9 Subclavian artery

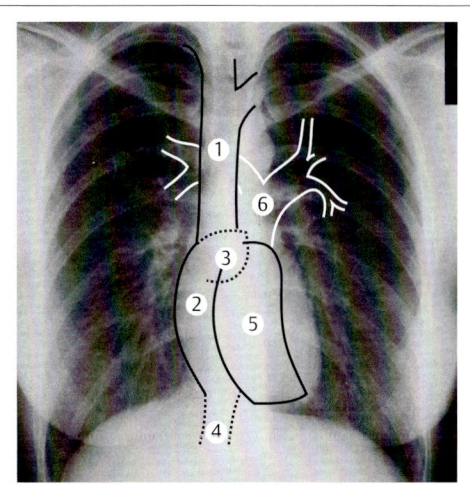

Fig. 11.2 Right cardiac structures and venous system:
1 Superior vena cava
2 Right atrium
3 Right atrial appendage
4 Inferior vena cava
5 Right ventricle
6 Pulmonary trunk

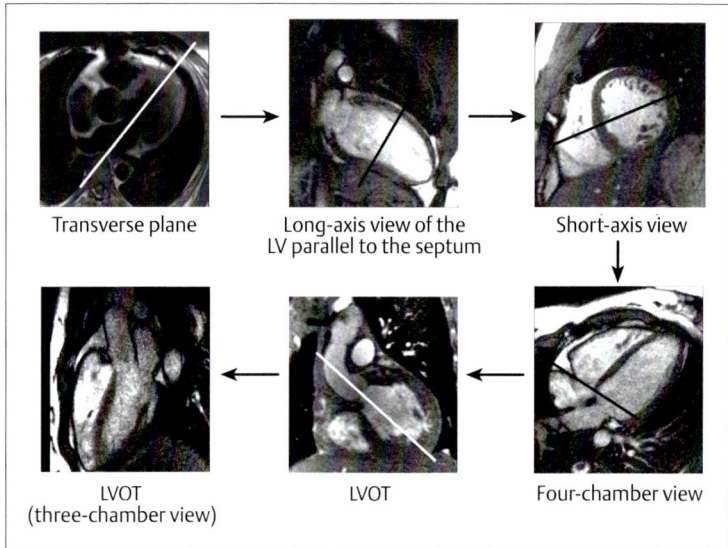

Transverse plane

Long-axis view of the LV parallel to the septum

Short-axis view

LVOT (three-chamber view)

LVOT

Four-chamber view

Fig. 11.3 Standard views for cardiac imaging. The lines indicate the angle and position of the next plane to be imaged.

Definition

▶ **Classification**

Cross-sectional modalities for cardiac imaging utilize standard views, which are applied in a similar manner in echocardiography, MRI, and ECG-synchronized multidetector CT.

The standard views used are:

  – Long-axis view of the RV or LV parallel to the interventricular septum.
  – Four-chamber view.
  – Short-axis view.
  – RVOT and LVOT (so-called "three-chamber view").

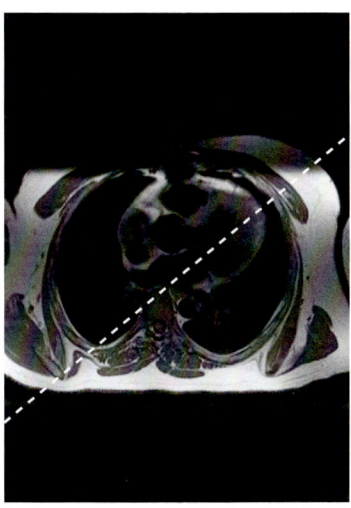

Fig. 11.4 T1-weighted MR image, TSE sequence. The line represents a longitudinal section through the left ventricle.

Fig. 11.5 Anatomy of the left ventricle (from Schünke M et al. *Thieme Atlas of Anatomy. Neck and Internal Organs*. Stuttgart: Thieme; 2006).

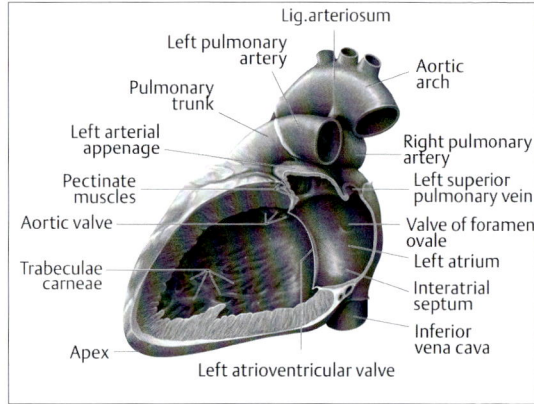

Fig. 11.6 Long-axis view of the left heart in a plane parallel to the septum. MR image, SSFP sequence in diastole.
* *   Left pulmonary artery
* +   Aortic arch with origin of the left carotid artery
* LA Left atrium
* x   Mitral valve
* LV Left ventricle

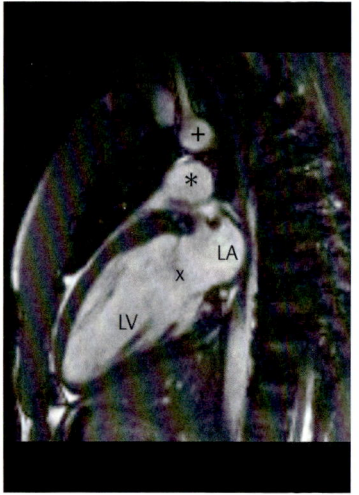

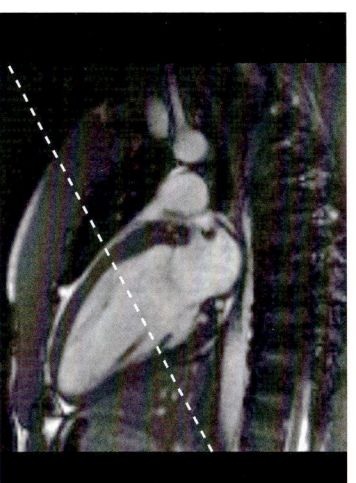

Fig. 11.7 Long-axis view of the left heart parallel to the plane of the septum. MR image, SSFP sequence in diastole. The line indicates the imaging plane of the short-axis view.

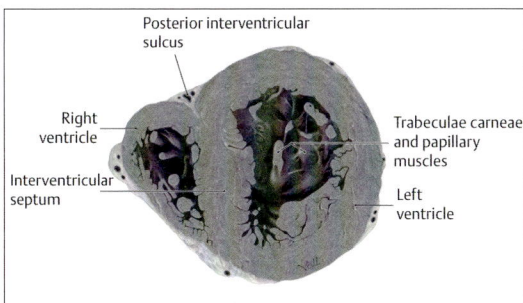

Posterior interventricular sulcus

Right ventricle

Interventricular septum

Trabeculae carneae and papillary muscles

Left ventricle

Fig. 11.8 Anatomy of the short-axis view of the heart (from Schünke M et al. *Thieme Atlas of Anatomy. Neck and Internal Organs*. Stuttgart: Thieme; 2006).

Fig. 11.9 Short-axis view through the right and left ventricles. Normal trabeculation is seen in both ventricles.
RV Right ventricle
LV Left ventricle

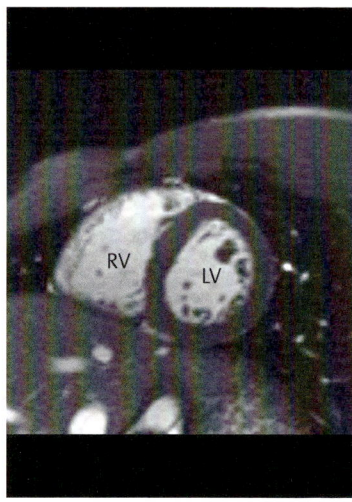

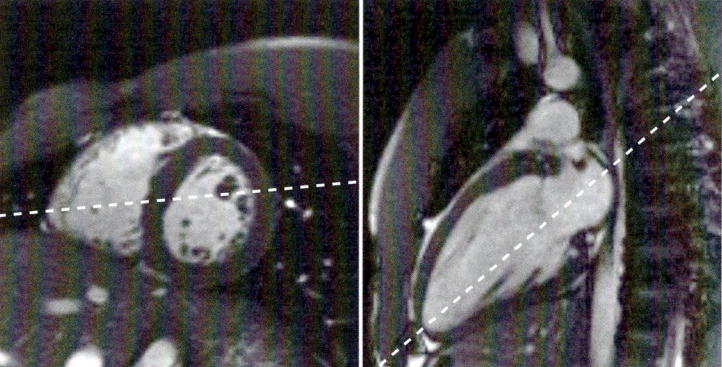

Fig. 11.10 Short- and long-axis views parallel to the plane of the septum. MR images, SSFP sequence in diastole. The line indicates the imaging plane for the four-chamber view.

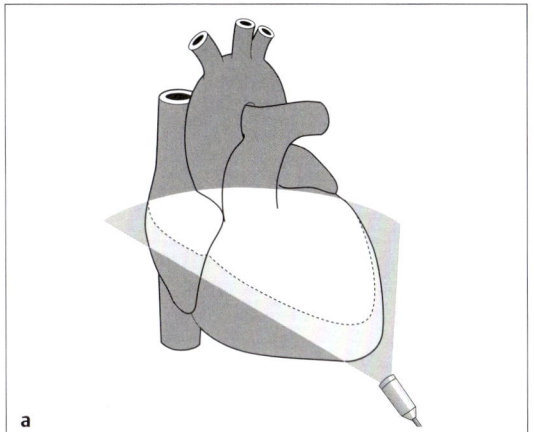

Fig. 11.11 a, b
Transducer position for imaging the heart in the four-chamber view (**a**) and the corresponding echocardiographic image (**b**).

RV   Right ventricle
LV   Left ventricle
TV   Tricuspid valve
MV   Mitral valve
RA   Right atrium
LA   Left atrium

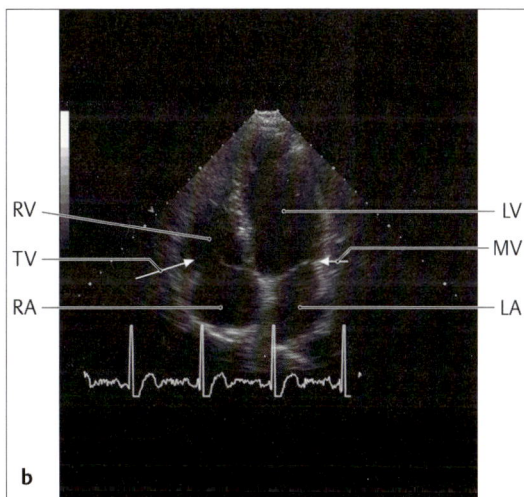

Fig. 11.12 Anatomy of the four-chamber view (from Schünke M et al. *Thieme Atlas of Anatomy. Neck and Internal Organs*. Stuttgart: Thieme; 2006).

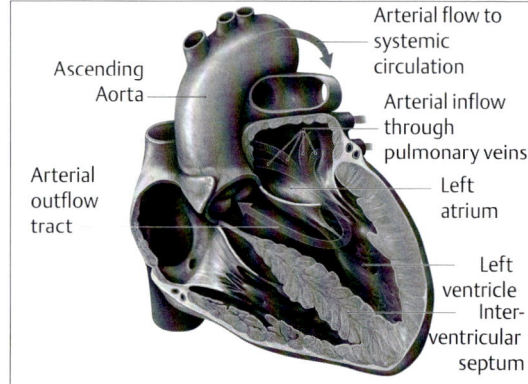

Ascending Aorta

Arterial outflow tract

Arterial flow to systemic circulation

Arterial inflow through pulmonary veins

Left atrium

Left ventricle

Inter-ventricular septum

Fig. 11.13 Four-chamber view. MR image, SSFP sequence in diastole, showing the atrioventricular unit of the right and left heart. Normal trabeculation is seen in both ventricles.

+ Crista terminalis, prominent part of the right atrial trabecular system
* Termination of the lower lobe veins

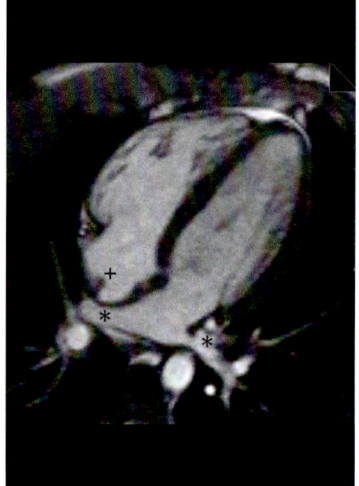

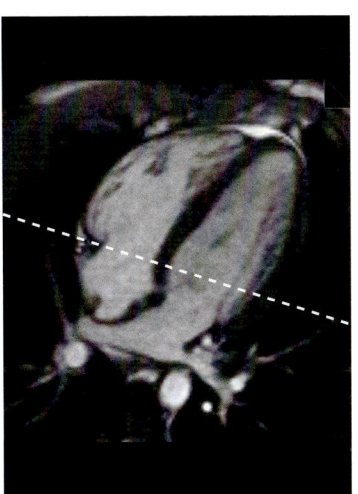

Fig. 11.14 Four-chamber view. MR image, SSFP sequence in diastole. The line indicates the plane of the LVOT.

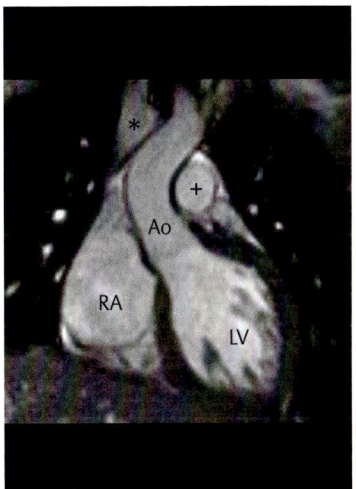

Fig. 11.15 LVOT. MR image, SSFP sequence in diastole.
+   Pulmonary trunk
*   Superior vena cava
Ao   Ascending aorta
RA   Right atrium
LV   Left ventricle

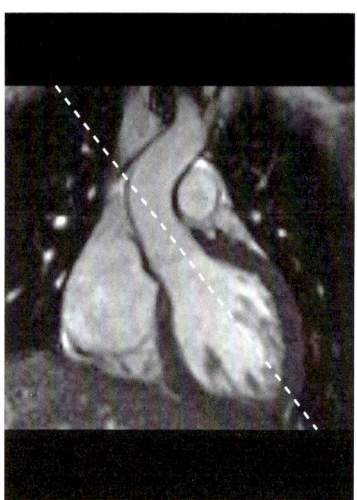

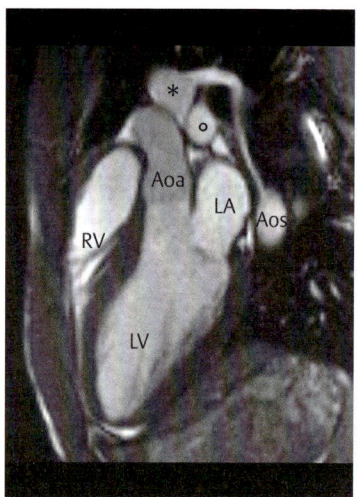

Fig. 11.16   LVOT. MR image, SSFP sequence in diastole. The line indicates the plane of the so-called "three-chamber view".

Fig. 11.17   LVOT. MR image, SSFP sequence in diastole.

*	Superior vena cava (with termination of azygos vein)
°	Right pulmonary artery
Aoa	Ascending aorta
Aos	Descending aorta
LA	Left atrium
RV	Right ventricle
LV	Left ventricle

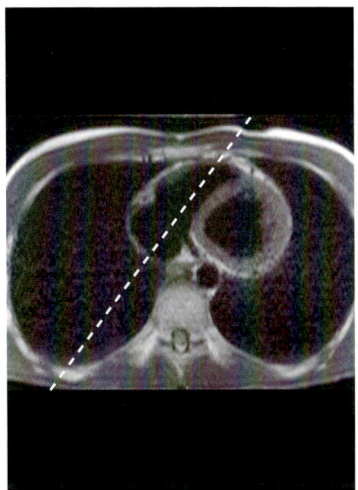

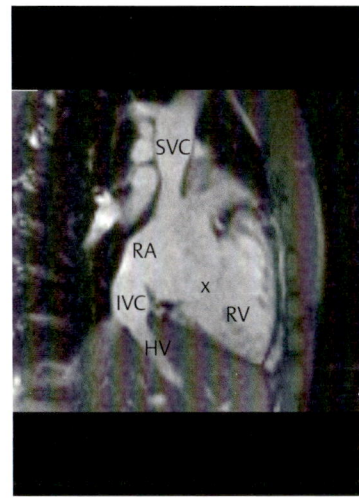

Fig. 11.18   T1-weighted MR image, TSE sequence. The line indicates a longitudinal section through the right ventricle.

Fig. 11.19   Long-axis view of the right heart parallel to the plane of the septum. MR image, SSFP sequence in diastole.

SVC   Superior vena cava
RA   Right atrium
RV   Right ventricle
x   Tricuspid valve
IVC   Inferior vena cava
HV   Hepatic vein

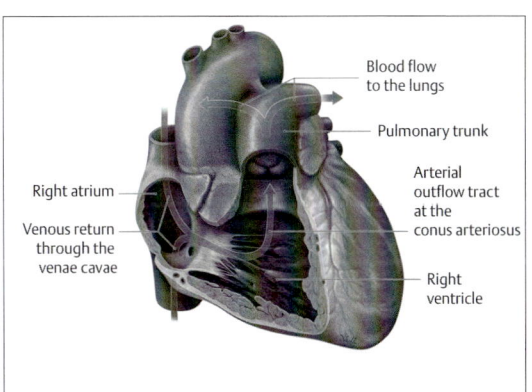

Blood flow to the lungs

Pulmonary trunk

Arterial outflow tract at the conus arteriosus

Right atrium

Venous return through the venae cavae

Right ventricle

Fig. 11.20   Anatomy of the right heart including the RVOT (from Schünke M et al. *Thieme Atlas of Anatomy. Neck and Internal Organs.* Stuttgart: Thieme; 2006).

Fig. 11.21 MR image, HASTE sequence. The lines indicate the RVOT plane.

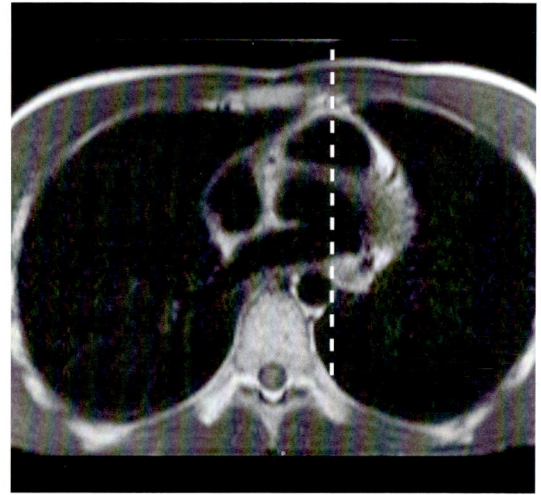

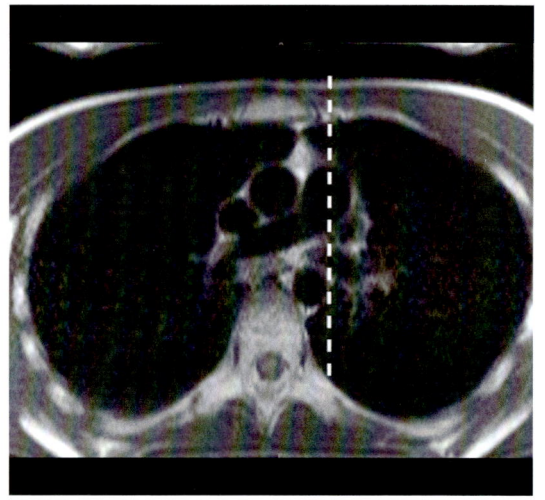

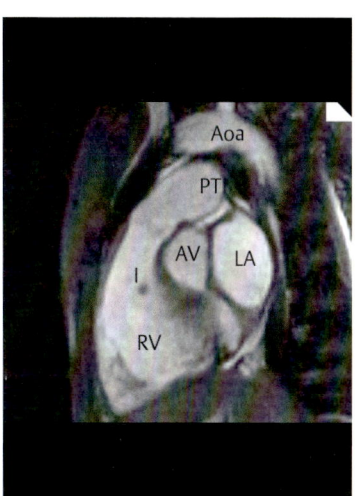

Fig. 11.22　RVOT. MR image, SSFP sequence in diastole.

Aoa Aortic arch
PT　Pulmonary trunk
AV　Aortic valve
I　　Infundibulum of the RVOT
LA　Left atrium
RV　Right ventricle

Table **1** **Normal measurements**

Parameter	Normal value
Diameter of ascending aorta	< 32 mm
Diameter of descending aorta	23–26 mm
Pulmonary artery	< 1.1 cm/m² body surface area
End-diastolic myocardial thickness:	
• LV septum	< 12 mm
• LV inferior wall	< 10 mm
• LV lateral wall	< 10 mm
• RV lateral wall	< 3 mm
End-diastolic short-axis diameter (midventricular):	
• LV	55 mm
• RV	26 mm
Ejection fraction (EF)	Approximately 50–75 % (different sources for echocardiography, MRI)
Cardiac index	2.4–2.6 L/m² body surface area

Table **2** **Absolute normal values** (range = mean value ± 2 SD)

Gradient echo				
	Men		**Women**	
	LV	**RV**	**LV**	**RV**
EDV (mL)	65–171	75–188	55–139	54–145
ESV (mL)	15–66	20–87	10–48	8–62
EF (%)	56–77	46–74	61–80	50–87
Weight (g)	119–190	–	79–141	–

SSFP				
	Men		**Women**	
	LV	**RV**	**LV**	**RV**
EDV (mL)	102–235	111–243	96–174	83–178
ESV (mL)	29–93	47–111	27–71	32–72
EF (%)	55–73	48–63	54–74	50–70
Weight (g)	85–181	–	66–114	–

Table **3**   **Normal values normalized to body surface area** (range = mean value ± 2 SD)

Gradient echo				
	Men		**Women**	
	LV	**RV**	**LV**	**RV**
EDV (mL)	34–84	42–89	36–77	36–80
ESV (mL)	8–33	12–41	7–27	6–35
EF (%)	56–77	46–74	61–80	50–87
Weight (g)	60–95	–	49–80	–

SSFP				
	Men		**Women**	
	LV	**RV**	**LV**	**RV**
EDV (mL)	53–112	58–114	56–99	48–103
ESV (mL)	15–45	25–53	14–40	18–42
EF (%)	55–73	48–63	54–74	50–70
Weight (g)	46–83	–	37–67	–

From: Guidelines for the use of magnetic resonance imaging in cardiac diagnosis (http://www.uni-wuerzburg.de/agherzdiagnostik/web/pdf/Leitlinien_MRT_190504.pdf)

References

Sandstede J, Lipke C, Beer M, Hofmann S, Pabst T, Kenn W, Neubauer S, Hahn D. Age- and gender-specific differences in left and right ventricular cardiac function and mass determined by cine magnetic resonance imaging. Eur Radiol 2000; 10: 438–442

Alfakih K, Plein S, Thiele H, Jones T, Ridgway JP, Sivananthan MU. Normal human left and right ventricular dimensions for MRI as assessed by turbo gradient echo and steady-state free precession imaging sequences. J Magn Reson Imaging 2003; 17: 323–329

AHA Classification of Myocardial Segments

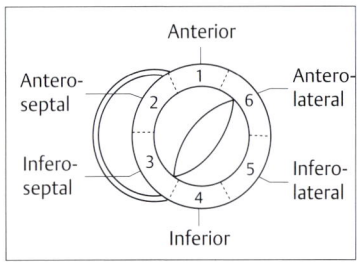

Fig. 12.1   Short-axis view, basal segments.

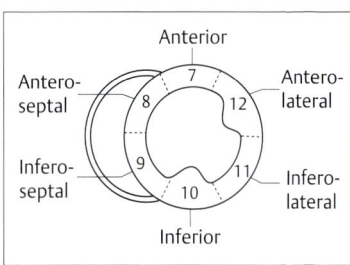

Fig. 12.2   Short-axis view, midventricular segments.

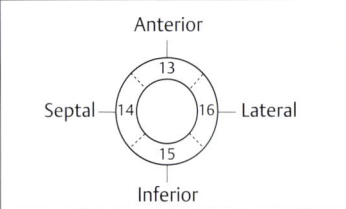

Fig. 12.3   Short-axis view, apical segments.

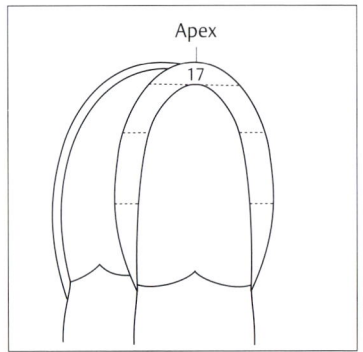

Fig. 12.4   Horizontal long-axis view (four-chamber view).

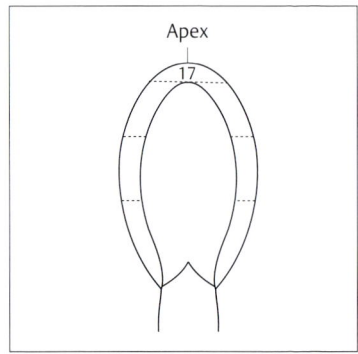

Fig. 12.5   Vertical long-axis view (two-chamber view).

Nomenclature for Sectional Cardiac Imaging

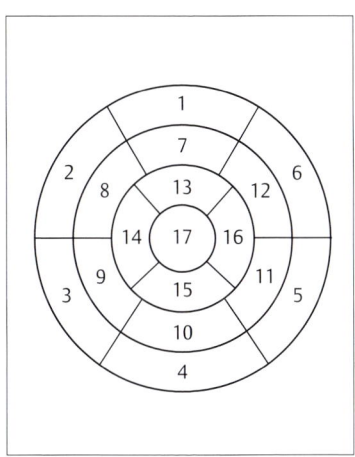

Fig. 12.6   The 17-segment model of the left ventricle:

1 Basal anterior
2 Basal anteroseptal
3 Basal inferoseptal
4 Basal inferior
5 Basal inferolateral
6 Basal anterolateral
7 Mid-anterior
8 Mid-anteroseptal
9 Mid-inferoseptal
10 Mid-inferior
11 Mid-inferolateral
12 Mid-anterolateral
13 Apical anterior
14 Apical septal
15 Apical inferior
16 Apical lateral
17 Apex

References

Cerqueira et al. Standardized myocardial segmentation and nomenclature for tomographic imaging of the heart: a statement for healthcare professionals from the Cardiac Imaging Committee of the Council on Clinical Cardiology of the American Heart Association. Circulation 2002; 105: 539–542

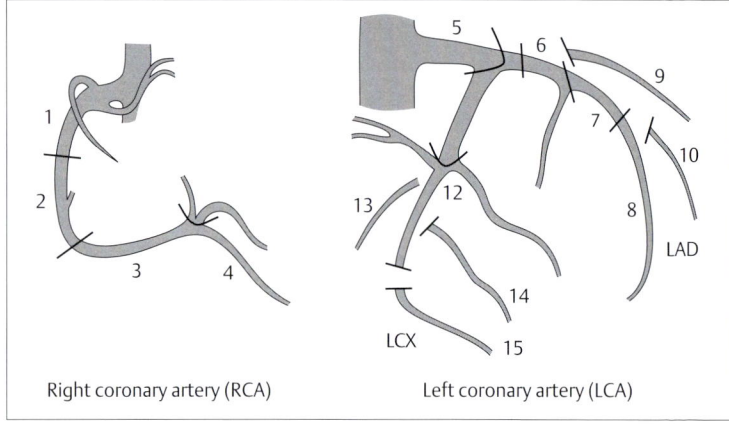

Fig. 12.7 Segments of the coronary arteries.
LAD Left anterior descending artery
LCX Circumflex branch

References

Austen WG et al. A reporting system on patients evaluated for coronary artery disease. Report of the Ad Hoc Committee for Grading of Coronary Artery Disease, Council on Cardiovascular Surgery, American Heart Association. Circulation 1975; 51: 5–40

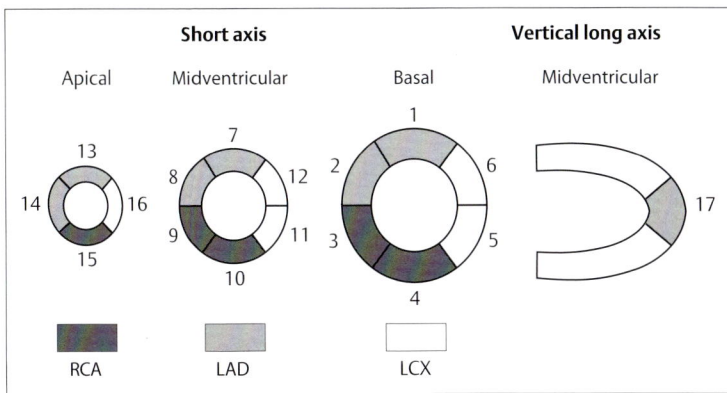

Fig. 12.8 Relationship of coronary territories to the 17-segment model.
RCA Right coronary artery
LAD Left anterior descending artery
LCX Circumflex branch of the LCA

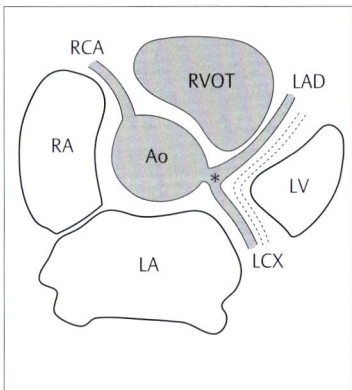

Fig. 12.9 Normal anatomy of the coronary origins.

RCA   Right coronary artery
RVOT   Right ventricular outflow tract
LAD   Left anterior descending artery
RA   Right atrium
Ao   Aorta
LV   Left ventricle
*   Left coronary artery
       (left main trunk)
LCX   Circumflex branch of LCA
LA   Left atrium

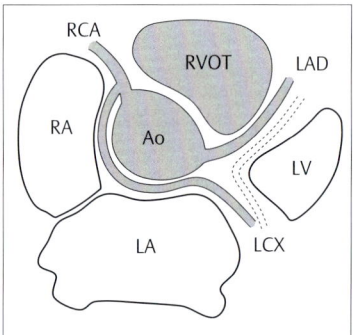

Fig. 12.10 Normal variant with the LCX arising from the RCA.

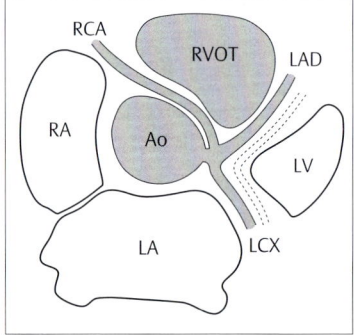

Fig. 12.11 Normal variant with the RCA arising from the LCA. Malignant variant in which the RCA runs between the aorta and RVOT.

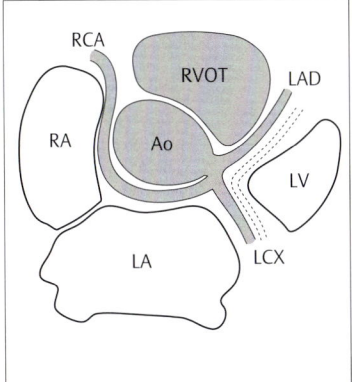

Fig. 12.12 Normal variant with the RCA arising from the LCA. Benign variant in which the RCA runs between the aorta and the LA and RA.

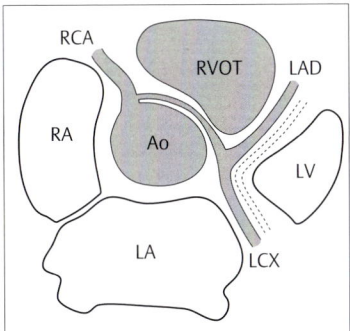

Fig. 12.13 Normal variant with the LCA arising from the RCA. Malignant variant in which the LCA runs between the aorta and RVOT.

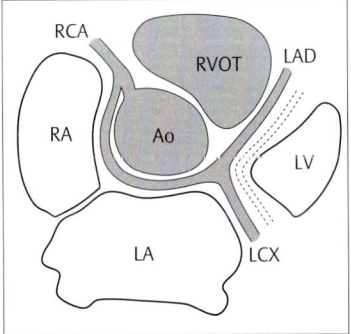

Fig. 12.14 Normal variant with the LCA arising from the RCA. Benign variant in which the LCA runs between the aorta and the LA and RA.

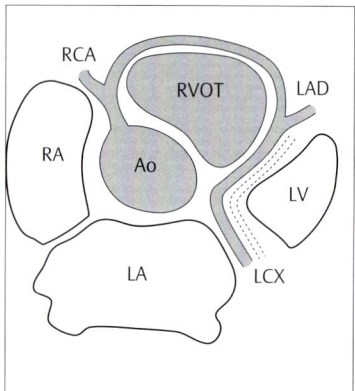

Fig. 12.15 Normal variant with the LCA arising from the RCA. Potentially malignant variant in which the LCA runs between the RVOT and LV.

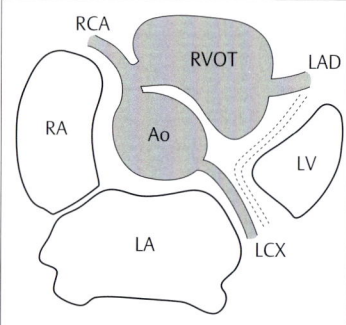

Fig. 12.16 Normal variant with the LAD arising from the RVOT and a coronary fistula between the RVOT and the RCA. The LCX arises directly from the aorta.

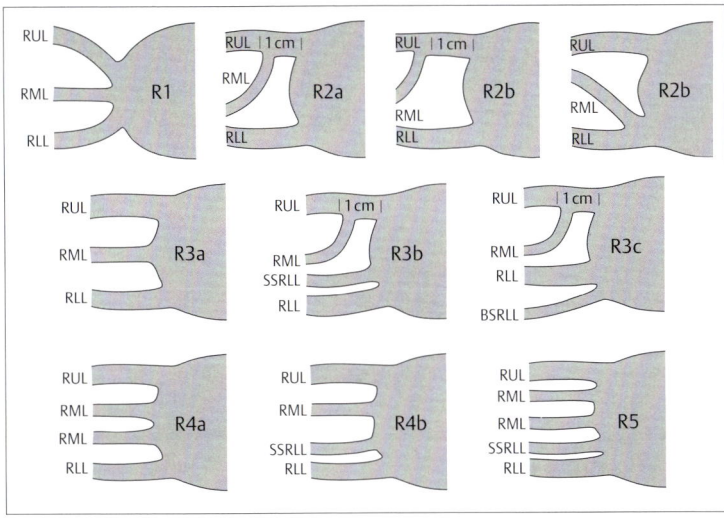

Fig. 12.17 Right pulmonary venous system.

RUL   Right upper lobe vein
RML   Right middle lobe vein
RLL   Right lower lobe vein
SSRLL   Right lower lobe vein, superior (apical) segment
BSRLL   Right lower lobe vein, basal segment

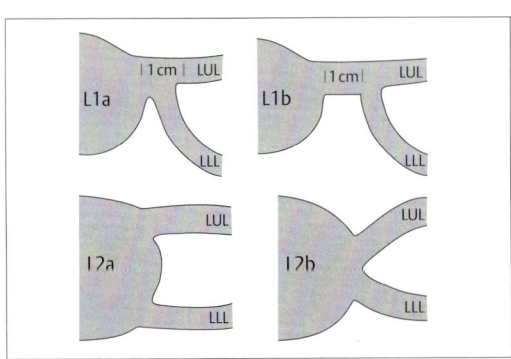

Fig. 12.18 Left pulmonary venous system.
LUL
Left upper lobe vein
LLL
Left lower lobe vein

References

Marom et al. Variations in Pulmonary Venous Drainage to the Left Atrium: Implications for Radiofrequency Ablation. Radiology 2004; 230: 824–829

Class I   No limitation of physical activity; ordinary activities do not cause symptoms.

Class II Mild limitation of physical activity; no symptoms at rest or with mild exertion.

Class III Marked limitation of physical activity; asymptomatic only at rest.

Class IV Symptomatic even at rest.

Primary cardiomyopathies

- DCM
- HCM/HOCM
- RCM
- ARVC

Secondary cardiomyopathies

- Inflammatory (autoimmune, viral)
- Toxic: alcohol, anthracyclines, cyclophosphamide, lithium, etc.
- Ischemic, valvular, hypertensive
- Induced by tachycardia
- Metabolic: hypo- or hyperthyroidism, uremia, diabetes mellitus, nutritional deficiency, electrolyte imbalance, etc.
- Systemic diseases: amyloidosis, lupus erythematosus, scleroderma, sarcoidosis, leukemias, rheumatoid arthritis, ankylosing spondylitis
- Neuromuscular diseases (Friedrich ataxia), muscular and myotonic dystrophies (Duchenne disease, Becker–Kiener disease, Curschmann–Steinert disease)
- Radiogenic
- Perinatal

Unclassified cardiomyopathies

- ILNC
- Fibroelastosis
- Systolic dysfunction with minimal dilatation
- Apical ballooning syndrome, identical with Tako–Tsubo syndrome
- Mitochondrial diseases

I	Global or regional dysfunction or structural changes	
	Major criteria	• Severe RV dilatation and reduction of the RV EF with little or no impairment of LV function • Localized RV aneurysms • Severe segmental RV dilatation
	Minor criteria	• Mild RV dilatation and reduction of the RV EF with normal LV function • Mild segmental RV dilatation • Regional RV hypokinesia • Trabecular hypertrophy*

II	Tissue characterization of the cardiac wall	
	Major criterion	• Fibrolipomatous transformation of the myocardium, detectable by myocardial biopsy

III	Repolarization abnormalities	
	Minor criterion	• Inverted T waves in right precordial leads (V_2–V_3) (age > 12 years, no RBBB)

IV	Depolarization and conduction abnormalities	
	Major criterion	• Epsilon waves or localized prolongation (> 110 ms) of the QRS complex in the right precordial leads (V_1–V_3)
	Minor criterion	• Late potentials

V	Arrhythmias	
	Major criteria	• Ventricular tachycardia with LBBB morphology (ECG, ambulatory ECG, stress ECG) • Frequent ventricular extrasystoles (> 1000/24h, ambulatory ECG)

VI	Family history	
	Major criterion	• Family history with anatomic confirmation (autopsy, surgery)
	Minor criteria	• Sudden cardiac death in family members < 35 years of age with suspected ARVC • Evidence of ARVC in family members based on clinical criteria

Diagnosis requires two major criteria, one major plus two minor criteria, or four minor criteria.
* Not considered a valid criterion by all authors.

Crawford Classification

Type I   Involves all of the descending thoracic aorta and proximal abdominal aorta, but without involving the renal or visceral arteries.

Type II   Involves all of the descending thoracic aorta and abdominal aorta.

Type III   Involves the middle and distal descending thoracic aorta and abdominolumbar aorta.

Type IV   Involves the thoracoabdominal junction and abdominolumbar aorta.

Type V   Involves only the abdominal aorta, including the renal arteries.

	Chest radio-graph	TTE, TEE	Invasive diagnos-tic pro-cedures	Multi-detec-tor CT	MRI	SPECT, PET
Morphology of cardiac chambers, pericardium	III	Ib	III	Ib	Ia	III
Morphology of coronary arteries	IV	IV	Ia	Ib	III	IV
Morphology of cardiac valves	IV	Ia	III	Ib	II	IV
Morphology of great vessels	III	III	III	Ia	Ia	IV
Qualitative myo-cardial function	IV	Ia	II	inv	Ib	III
Quantitative myo-cardial function	IV	Ib	III	inv	Ia	III
Qualitative valve function	IV	Ia	II	inv	II	IV
Quantitative valve function	IV	Ia	III	inv	II	IV
Myocardial perfusion	IV	inv	IV	inv	Ib	Ia
Myocardial metabo-lism	IV	IV	IV	IV	inv	Ia
Myocardial viability	IV	III*	III	inv	Ia	Ib
Structural tissue changes	IV	IV	Ia†	III	Ib	III‡
Volume and flow assessment	IV	Ib	Ia	IV	Ib	IV
Pressure relationships	IV	II	Ia	IV	III	IV
Impulse conduction	IV	IV	Ia	inv	inv	III

Ia   First choice modality.
Ib   Alternative to Ia as a first-line study.
II   Often used and well established but provides information that can also be obtained with other modalities.
III   Used occasionally, provides information that is generally obtained with other modalities.
IV   Does not provide clinically relevant information.
inv Investigative, probably yields relevant information, still undergoing trials.
Invasive diagnostic procedures = cardiac catheterization studies including coronary angiography and electrophysiologic test procedures.
CT, computed tomography; MRI, magnetic resonance imaging; TTE, transthoracic echocardiography; TEE, transesophageal echocardiography; SPECT, single photon emission computed tomography; PET, positron emission tomography.
*   Stress echocardiography; † myocardial biopsy; ‡ of limited usefulness.

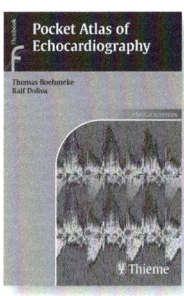
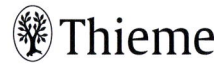

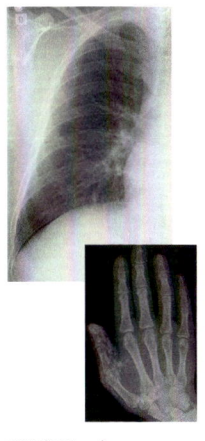
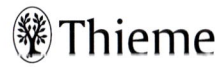